CONTRACEPTION
MADE EASY

CONTRACEPTION
MADE EASY
THIRD EDITION

LAURA PERCY

Consultant in Community Reproductive and Sexual Health
Newcastle upon Tyne, UK

and

DIANA MANSOUR

Consultant in Community Gynaecology and Reproductive Healthcare
New Croft Centre, Newcastle upon Tyne, UK

Scion

© **Scion Publishing Ltd, 2023**

ISBN 9781914961342

Third edition published 2023

Second edition published 2020

First revised edition published 2016

First edition published 2015

A CIP catalogue record for this book is available from the British Library.

Scion Publishing Limited

The Old Hayloft, Vantage Business Park, Bloxham Road, Banbury OX16 9UX, UK

www.scionpublishing.com

Important Note from the Publisher

The information contained within this book was obtained by Scion Publishing Ltd from sources believed by us to be reliable. However, while every effort has been made to ensure its accuracy, no responsibility for loss or injury whatsoever occasioned to any person acting or refraining from action as a result of information contained herein can be accepted by the authors or publishers.

Readers are reminded that medicine is a constantly evolving science and while the authors and publishers have ensured that all dosages, applications and practices are based on current indications, there may be specific practices which differ between communities. You should always follow the guidelines laid down by the manufacturers of specific products and the relevant authorities in the country in which you are practising.

Although every effort has been made to ensure that all owners of copyright material have been acknowledged in this publication, we would be pleased to acknowledge in subsequent reprints or editions any omissions brought to our attention.

Registered names, trademarks, etc. used in this book, even when not marked as such, are not to be considered unprotected by law.

Illustrations by Hilary Strickland

Typeset by Evolution Design & Digital Ltd (Kent)

Printed in the UK

Last digit is the print number: 10 9 8 7 6 5 4 3 2 1

Contents

Foreword to the second edition

I was delighted to be asked to write this Foreword, because in the author team there is such an excellent combination of clinical acumen and experience of writing and publishing. I have always appreciated Diana's understanding of the evidence and research behind her management. Laura was the first winner of the Anne Szarewski Journal Memorial Award for clinical innovation.

Diana and Laura have brought together current FSRH guidance, NICE guidelines and clinical practice in a concise form for easy reference. I was particularly impressed by the coverage of contraception for special groups (*Chapter 3*) and unplanned pregnancy (*Chapter 15*). A summary of the UK Medical Eligibility Criteria (UKMEC) as an Appendix is very useful. This book genuinely is 'contraception made easy'.

Concise and practical, this book is ideal to have at hand wherever contraceptive care is being provided: in primary or community care, or in a secondary care setting. Alternatively you may wish simply to update your knowledge. Enjoy!

Dr Asha Kasliwal, President FSRH

About the authors

Dr Laura Percy qualified as a Consultant in Community Sexual and Reproductive Healthcare, and is currently an Associate Editor of *BMJ Sexual & Reproductive Health*. She was the winner of the inaugural Anne Szarewski Journal Memorial Award, and has published several articles on Contraception and Women's Health. She completed her MBBS from the University of Newcastle upon Tyne in 2006, began working in contraception in 2008. She has an MSc in Health Education and Health Promotion, and a BSc in Human Biology from King's College, London. Laura is a qualified psychosexual therapist and has a special interest in this area. She is also very interested in the provision of medical information to the public and professionals, with a particular emphasis on sexual health. Information provision and dissemination is currently the main focus of her work.

Dr Diana Mansour is a Consultant in Community Gynaecology and Reproductive Healthcare in Newcastle upon Tyne, UK. She has been an Associate Clinical Lecturer at Newcastle University since 1997. In addition Dr Mansour was the Senior Vice President at the Faculty of Sexual and Reproductive Healthcare in the UK and Past Chair of the FSRH Clinical Effectiveness Committee. She sits on the Steering Group and Guideline Development Group for the UK Medical Eligibility Criteria for Contraceptive Use.

Dr Mansour was the first accredited subspecialty trainee in Community Gynaecology and Reproductive Healthcare of the Royal College of Obstetricians and Gynaecologists.

She is first author to over 90 peer-reviewed publications. Her areas of expertise include acceptability of contraceptive methods, non-contraceptive benefits of contraception, development of long-term methods of contraception, changes in health service provision, medical management of heavy menstrual bleeding and management of the menopause.

Abbreviations

ART	antiretroviral therapy
BMD	bone mineral density
BMI	body mass index
BNF	*British National Formulary*
CHC	combined hormonal contraception
CIN	cervical intraepithelial neoplasia
COC	combined oral contraceptive
CTP	combined transdermal patch
CVE	cardiovascular event
CVR	combined vaginal ring
DMPA	depot medroxyprogesterone acetate
DVT	deep vein thrombosis
EC	emergency contraception
EVA	electronic vacuum aspiration
FPA	Family Planning Association
FSH	follicle-stimulating hormone
hCG	human chorionic gonadotrophin
HFI	hormone-free interval
HMB	heavy menstrual bleeding
IBD	inflammatory bowel disease
IMB	intermenstrual bleeding
IMP	implant

IUC	intrauterine contraceptive
IUD	intrauterine device
IUS	intrauterine system
IVF	*in vitro* fertilization
LAM	lactational amenorrhoea method
LARC	long-acting reversible contraception
LH	luteinizing hormone
LNG	levonorgestrel
MI	myocardial infarction
MIV	minimally invasive vasectomy
MSM	men who are gay, bisexual or have sex with other men
MVA	manual vacuum aspiration
NET-EN	norethisterone enanthate
NICE	National Institute for Health and Care Excellence
NSAID	non-steroidal anti-inflammatory drug
NSV	no-scalpel vasectomy
PCB	post-coital bleeding
PE	pulmonary embolism
PEP	post-exposure prophylaxis
PID	pelvic inflammatory disease
POP	progestogen-only pill
PrEP	pre-exposure prophylaxis
RCOG	Royal College of Obstetricians and Gynaecologists
STI	sexually transmitted infection
UKMEC	UK Medical Eligibility Criteria
UPA	ulipristal acetate
UPSI	unprotected sexual intercourse
VTE	venous thromboembolism

Chapter 1
Introduction

1.1 Introduction

This short book provides up-to-date information, often in note form, about the commonly used contraceptive methods available in high resource countries and is aimed at healthcare professionals working in primary, community and secondary services. The book's content is based on guidance from the Faculty of Sexual and Reproductive Healthcare's Clinical Effectiveness Unit and the National Institute for Health and Care Excellence. References will appear at the end of each chapter when specific studies or reviews are mentioned.

Chapter 2, covering the consultation, explores the necessary points to discuss when seeing couples about contraception, including their ideas, concerns and expectations. *Chapter 3* looks in more detail at the provision of contraception to special groups such as young people and those with learning difficulties. Each method will then be examined in turn, with information identifying potential users of the method, how it works, its efficacy, the advantages and disadvantages, how to start and stop the methods (where appropriate) plus the management of troublesome side-effects. The book concludes with two chapters on screening women for asymptomatic sexually transmitted infections (STI) and managing unplanned pregnancies.

1.2 Unplanned pregnancy

Keeping up to date in this field is difficult, especially when contraception is not your special interest. Yet men and women will seek advice from approachable healthcare staff who are non-judgemental and can give non-directional support. Hopefully being better prepared will help couples plan their pregnancies. However, at the current time it is estimated that almost 50% of pregnancies worldwide are unplanned. One in three women from high resource countries experiences an abortion during their lifetime, with a third requiring a repeat procedure.

Over 80% of abortions take place in women aged 20 or over, not the teenagers that are so often vilified. Free provision of contraception has had little effect on the abortion rate in England and Wales (*Figures 1.1–1.3*), with at least 60% of women using a contraceptive method at the time of the abortion. However, the most commonly cited methods are oral contraceptives or condoms, which require correct and consistent use. This high number of unplanned pregnancies may reflect poor contraceptive knowledge in the population. There may be issues related to funding of contraceptive services in primary and community care which limit access to and availability of contraceptive choice. Time pressures during consultations reduce the ability to explore fears and concerns surrounding some methods. This can result in couples choosing a contraceptive that fails to fit their lifestyle, for example an inability to adhere to daily regimens, leading to high typical failure rates for pills, condoms and natural methods when compared with perfect use (*Table 1.1*).

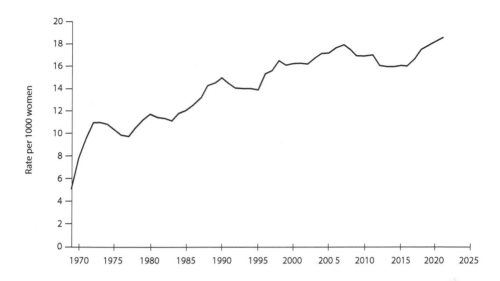

Figure 1.1 Age-standardized abortion rate per 1000 women aged 15–44, England and Wales 1970 to 2021.

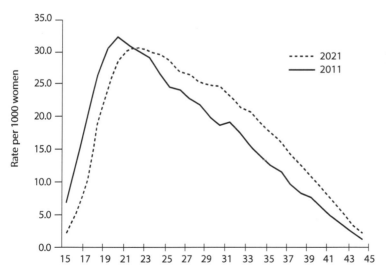

Figure 1.2 Abortion rate per 1000 women by single year of age, England and Wales, 2011 and 2021.

Table 1.1 Summary table of contraceptive efficacy – percentage of women experiencing an unintended pregnancy during the first year of typical and perfect use of contraception, and the percentage continuing use of that contraceptive at the end of the first year of use

Contraceptive method	Women experiencing an unintended pregnancy within the first year of use (%)		Women continuing use at 1 year (%)
	Typical use	Perfect use	
No method	85	85	
Spermicides	21	16	42
Fertility awareness-based methods	15		47
Simplified calendar method	12	5	
Standard days method	12	5	
Two day method	14	4	
Ovulation method	23	3	
Symptothermal method	2	0.4	
Withdrawal	20	4	46
Sponge	17	12	36
Parous women	27	20	
Nulliparous women	14	9	
Condom			
Female	21	5	41
Male	13	2	43
Diaphragm	17	16	57
Combined pill and progestogen-only pill	7	0.3	67
Evra patch	7	0.3	67
NuvaRing	7	0.3	67
Depo-Provera	4	0.2	56
Intrauterine contraception			
TT380 Slimline/T-Safe 380A QL	0.8	0.6	78
Jaydess (13.5 mg LNG)	0.4	0.3	
Kyleena (19.5 mg LNG)	0.2	0.2	
Levosert (52 mg LNG)	0.1	0.1	
Mirena (52 mg LNG)	0.1	0.1	80
Nexplanon	0.1	0.1	89
Female sterilization	0.5	0.5	100
Male sterilization	0.15	0.10	100
Adapted from Trussell (2018).			

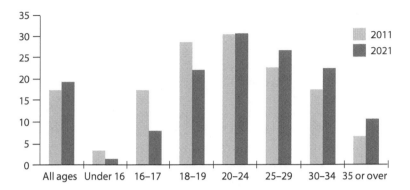

Figure 1.3 Abortion rate per 1000 women by age, England and Wales, 2011 and 2021.

1.3 Provision of contraceptive services

Political commitment to invest in contraceptive choice and easily accessible services is essential. Effective provision of, and access to, contraception improves the health of women and children. Investing in this area of healthcare is cost-effective; over a ten-year period, for every £1 spent on providing contraception in the UK, £9 from the public purse is saved.

1.4 UK Medical Eligibility Criteria for contraception

Sixteen contraceptive methods are available free at the point of access in the UK and these include:
- emergency contraception
- combined oral contraceptives (COCs), patches, and vaginal rings
- progestogen-only pills (POPs)
- progestogen-only injectables and implants (DMPA and IMP)
- copper intrauterine contraceptives (IUDs)
- levonorgestrel intrauterine systems (IUSs)
- diaphragms, cervical caps
- male and female condoms
- natural fertility awareness advice/kits/apps
- male and female sterilization.

Healthcare professionals may be fully aware of the contraceptive options available to couples but have concerns if certain medical conditions are present. This could deny women at greatest risk of maternal morbidity and mortality highly effective birth control methods. The UK Medical Eligibility Criteria (UKMEC) for contraceptive use is based on guidance from the World Health Organization and has been modified for use in the UK, guiding health professionals towards safer prescribing. The role of the UKMEC is to consider the safety of a method of contraception but not its efficacy with regard to medical conditions and patient characteristics. (See *Appendix* for full details of the UKMEC).

The UKMEC is a comprehensive reference tool for those prescribing contraception. The recommendations within it are based on current research, evidence and expert opinion. It includes four categories of risk applicable to contraceptive methods and these are shown in *Table 1.2*, but can be simply viewed as follows:
- UK Category 1 – no restriction for use
- UK Category 2 – can generally be used but with careful follow-up
- UK Category 3 – not usually recommended but may be used after expert clinical judgement and/or referral to a contraceptive specialist
- UK Category 4 – use poses an unacceptable health risk.

In certain cases, initiation (I) of a contraceptive method is classified differently from continuation (C) of a method:
- initiation – starting a method of contraception by a woman with a specific medical condition
- continuation – continuing with the method already being used by a woman who develops a new medical condition.

In this table, the numbers always refer to the UK Category of risk and in some instances the risk level is different at initiation (I) and continuation (C). The UKMEC should be used as a guide but should not replace clinical judgement. For a summary of the UKMEC see *Appendix*.

Table 1.2 Four categories of risk applicable to contraceptive methods

UK category	Hormonal contraception, IUDs and barrier methods
1	A condition for which there is no restriction for the use of the contraceptive method.
2	A condition where the advantages of using the method generally outweigh the theoretical or proven risks.
3	A condition where the theoretical or proven risks usually outweigh the advantages of using the method. Provision of this method requires expert clinical judgement and/or referral to a specialist contraceptive provider because use of the method is not usually recommended unless other methods are not available or not acceptable.
4	A condition which represents an unacceptable health risk if the contraceptive method is used.

Adapted from the Faculty of Sexual and Reproductive Healthcare's UKMEC for contraception, with kind permission.

References

Department of Health (2023) *Abortion Statistics, England and Wales: 2021* [www.gov.uk/government/statistics/abortion-statistics-for-england-and-wales-2021/abortion-statistics-england-and-wales-2021 – accessed May 2023]

NICE (2014) Clinical guideline 30: *Long-acting reversible contraception* (updated July 2019) [www.nice.org.uk/guidance/cg30 – accessed May 2023]

Public Health England (2018) *Contraception: economic analysis estimation of the return on investment (ROI) for publicly funded contraception in England* [https://assets.publishing.service.gov.uk/government/uploads/system/uploads/attachment_data/file/730292/contraception_return_on_investment_report.pdf – accessed May 2023]

Trussell J. (2018) *Contraceptive efficacy*. In Hatcher, R.A. *et al. Contraceptive Technology*, 21st edition. New York, NY: Ardent Media. [https://contraceptivetechnology.org/wp-content/uploads/2022/10/Contraceptive-Failure-Rates.pdf – accessed May 2023]

UKMEC (2016) *UK Medical Eligibility Criteria for Contraceptive Use* [www.fsrh.org/ukmec – accessed May 2023]

Chapter 2

The contraception consultation

2.1 Introduction

The primary aim of the contraception consultation is to enable women to choose the most suitable and acceptable method of birth control for their lifestyle.

A detailed history will help in determining which of the sixteen available methods can be used safely. Furthermore, taking a careful sexual history provides an opportunity for risk assessment, screening for infection and health promotion.

A variety of consultation models exist. They act as aids to help in the development of consultation skills with the aim of generating a patient-centred discussion. Their emphasis is on shared decision making and active participation by both parties. The contraception consultation could be based around any of these models. We suggest the Calgary–Cambridge approach, illustrated in *Figure 2.1*, which offers a useful framework and will be used throughout this book to provide a basic structure for the consultation.

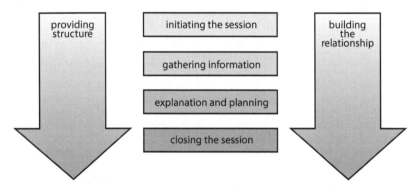

Figure 2.1 Calgary–Cambridge consultation model.

2.2 Initiating the session

This can be divided into two components:
- Establishing initial rapport:
  - greeting the patient
  - introducing yourself.
- Identifying the reason for the consultation:
  - this is ideally undertaken through the use of open questions, for example, *"How can I help you today?"* or *"What would you like to discuss?"*
  - the answers may range from specific requests for a particular method of contraception to the more complex "I need contraception but everything I have tried causes me problems"
  - supporting patients to set the agenda focuses the consultation on the patient's needs and helps to establish rapport.

2.3 Gathering information

- Explore the patient's narrative through a progression from open to closed questions, with active listening.
- An empathetic, non-judgemental approach with appropriate use of summaries or clarifying statements is often beneficial.
- Enable the patient to indicate their ideas, concerns and expectations.
  - **Ideas** – methods of contraception they have considered or previously used; this may include asking about problems encountered with previous methods, why previous contraception was stopped, or what they liked or disliked about previous choices.
  - **Concerns** – for example, worries about side-effects or perceptions about particular methods; this also provides an opportunity to myth bust about contraceptive methods, for example, "pills" cause weight gain and intrauterine devices or systems cannot be used by women who have not had children.
  - **Expectations** – for example, true efficacy, acceptable side-effects.
  - Future plans – would becoming pregnant be a disaster, are there plans to start a family or have another child in the near future?
- By using this approach one can easily determine acceptable methods and those which would be less likely to suit an individual (see *Figure 2.2*).
- Subsequently, a review of a patient's past medical, medication, family and social histories can be used to assess medical suitability for various methods. A detailed summary of the medical history is outlined in *Box 2.1*.
  - This history can be used to determine if there are any contraindications to a particular method of contraception through the application of the UK Medical Eligibility Criteria (UKMEC) – see *Appendix*.
  - A brief review of medical history is often of benefit at each new attendance to ensure circumstances have not changed. If a new medical condition has developed or medication has been initiated or changed, continuation of a patient's chosen method may be inappropriate.

2.4 Explanation and planning

This section of the consultation ideally incorporates the provision of information about available methods including mechanism of action, efficacy, risks, side-effects, and advantages and disadvantages, leading to a shared decision about which method to commence.

- There are a number of possible approaches to take to achieve this:
  - Each method could be briefly discussed followed by a more detailed discussion of those the patient is most interested in; this can be very time-consuming.
  - Alternatively, a good starting point could be to discuss the methods the patient is interested in and then expand on others as needed.
  - Some clinicians start by asking the patient what they know already about individual methods and then build on this foundation. For example, many patients are using online tools such as the 'My contraception tool'

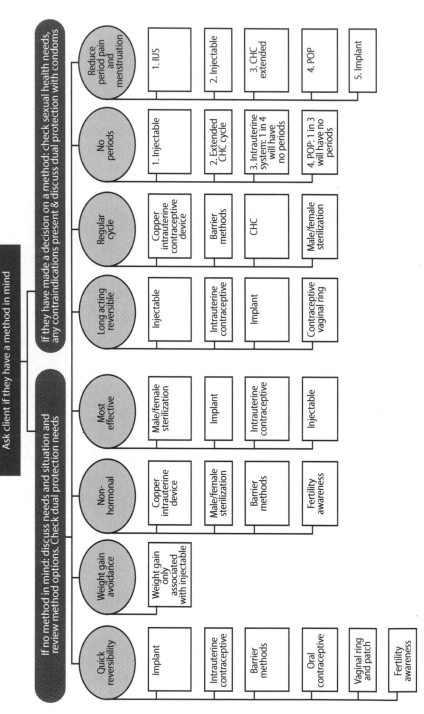

Figure 2.2 Decision tree for contraceptive options.

(www.brook.org.uk/our-services/start-my-contraception-tool) or the NHS 'Which method of contraception suits me?' (www.nhs.uk/conditions/contraception/which-method-suits-me).

○ Finally, you could ask an open question such as *"Apart from preventing a pregnancy, what else would you like your contraceptive method to achieve or help with, such as, to help with period pain or skin problems?"*.

Box 2.1 Medical history taking in a contraceptive consultation

Age

Gynaecological history

Menstrual cycle details
- Last menstrual period (normal or not)
- Length of cycle (longest and shortest)
- Regularity
- Bleeding irregularities – presence of intermenstrual bleeding (IMB) or post-coital bleeding (PCB), their frequency, duration, and associated symptoms such as pain
- Heavy menstrual bleeding (HMB) or dysmenorrhoea

History of gynaecological conditions
- Ovarian cysts
- Endometriosis
- Pelvic infection

Cervical screening history, if appropriate

Obstetric history
- Previous pregnancies – planned and unplanned
- Number of children, mode of delivery and problems during pregnancy
- Breastfeeding
- Miscarriages
- Ectopic pregnancies
- Abortions

Sexual history
- Any sexual problems?
- Symptoms of sexually transmitted infection (STI) including dysuria, change in vaginal discharge, abdominal pain, skin changes/rash

- Number of sexual partners in last 6 months/recent change in partner
- Condom use

Past medical history (including but not limited to)
- Epilepsy
- Diabetes
- Hypertension
- Cardiovascular disease
- Venous thromboembolism
- Cerebrovascular disease
- Migraine with or without aura

Medication
- Liver enzyme inducers, e.g. carbamazepine, St. John's wort
- Anti-epileptics
- Herbal remedies/over-the-counter medications

Allergies

Family history – including age at diagnosis and relation to patient
- Myocardial infarction (MI)
- Cardiovascular event (CVE)
- Venous thromboembolism (VTE)
- Breast cancer
- Ovarian cancer

Social history
- Smoking – amount per week
- Alcohol usage – amount per week
- Domestic violence – physical or emotional
- Female genital mutilation
- Religious and/or cultural beliefs – may affect contraceptive options

- Ideally information should be provided in small chunks, with regular checks of understanding and at a level appropriate to the individual attending the clinic.
- Practically, the most important aspects to ensure an individual understands about their chosen method are:
  - How to use the method, including missed doses and circumstances when a method will not be effective; for example, vomiting when taking the COC.
  - How long before it becomes effective.
  - Its benefits, risks and side-effects.
  - Safety-netting to ensure that individuals know when to seek help.
  - Provision of high quality information, such as links to the NHS website (www.nhs.uk/conditions/contraception) can be useful for women to have as a reference at home.
- When discussing and commencing contraception it is important to assess for the need for emergency contraception provision (see *Chapter 13*).
- There are a number of options when starting to use a contraceptive, including:
  - Waiting until an individual's next period before starting contraception, at which time the contraceptive method is immediately effective.
  - 'Quick starting' is starting contraception at the time a woman requests it. All methods of contraception can be quick started at any point in the menstrual cycle, providing pregnancy can be reasonably excluded. Criteria to aid in this exclusion are outlined in *Box 2.2*. Women who choose to quick start when pregnancy cannot be excluded are advised to undertake a high sensitivity pregnancy test. If this is negative they can commence either combined

---

Box 2.2 Criteria for reasonably excluding pregnancy (FSRH, 2017)

Healthcare practitioners can be reasonably certain that a woman is not currently pregnant if any one or more of the following criteria are met **and** there are no symptoms or signs of pregnancy:

- No intercourse since the start of her last normal (natural) menstrual period, since childbirth, abortion, miscarriage, ectopic pregnancy or uterine evacuation for gestational trophoblastic disease
- Correct and consistent use of a reliable method of contraception (barrier methods of contraception can be considered reliable providing they have been used consistently and correctly for every episode of intercourse)

- The woman attends within the first 5 days of the onset of a normal (natural) menstrual period
- She is less than 21 days postpartum (non-breastfeeding women)
- She is fully breastfeeding, amenorrhoeic AND less than 6 months postpartum
- She is within the first 5 days after abortion, miscarriage, ectopic pregnancy or uterine evacuation for gestational trophoblastic disease
- She has not had intercourse for >21 days AND has a negative high sensitivity urine pregnancy test (able to detect hCG levels of around 20 IU/ml)

hormonal contraception, the progestogen-only pill, implant or injection. When discussing quick starting it is also important to assess the potential need for emergency contraception and the impact of the provision of emergency contraception on an individual's chosen method (see *Chapter 13*). With all quick starting methods, additional precautions such as condoms or abstinence will be needed until the quick started method becomes effective. *Box 2.3* contains a checklist for quick starting contraception if a pregnancy cannot be excluded.

○ Using a bridging method of contraception, whereby one method of contraception is chosen in the short term until the requested method of contraception can be provided. Bridging may be required because an individual's chosen method is not available or is not suitable for quick starting; for example, using the POP until pregnancy can be excluded or until an appointment can be arranged to undertake an IUS fitting. This may require explanation as to where an individual can obtain their chosen contraceptive if it is not available in your service/practice.

Box 2.3 Checklist for quick starting when there is a potential risk of very early pregnancy

- Explain why pregnancy cannot be excluded
- Discuss options including delay in beginning contraception until pregnancy has been excluded and quick starting contraception immediately, with reference to ongoing potential risk of pregnancy from further episodes of unprotected sexual intercourse
- Advise the woman that quick starting is outside the product licence for many methods but supported by the FSRH
- Reassure that the vast majority of evidence suggests fetal exposure to contraceptive hormones does not negatively impact pregnancy outcomes
- Determine the need for EC: if LNG-EC is administered, CHC, POP, IMP (and DMPA) can be quick started immediately; however, if UPA-EC is administered then the individual needs to wait 120 hours before quick starting COC, POP, IMP (and DMPA)
- CHC (except co-cyprindiol), POP and implant can be quick started and barrier methods or abstinence are needed until the quick started method becomes effective
- DMPA can be quick started if other methods are not suitable or accepted (barrier methods or abstinence are needed until this method becomes effective)
- A copper IUD can be quick started if the indications for emergency contraception are met
- Indicate that a pregnancy test is indicated 21 days after the last episode of UPSI or 28 days after quick starting (to identify pregnancy which may have occurred in the week before the contraceptive method became effective)

- Discussion regarding risk of STI, advice on safer sexual practices including additional use of condoms, and the offer of STI testing are important components of a contraception choices consultation.
  - Offer chlamydia and gonorrhoea testing through self-taken vaginal swabs along with blood tests for HIV and syphilis (see *Chapter 14* for more details).
  - Provide information about local condom distribution schemes.
- The contraception consultation provides an opportunity to make enquiry about a history and/or potential risk of female genital mutilation (FGM). If the occurrence of FGM or potential risk is identified, national and local pathways should be followed.

EXAMPLE

A 21 year old woman with a history of migraine attends requesting contraception.

Consider which questions you need to ask and which contraceptive options would be appropriate.

1. It is important to determine the nature of the migraine – is it migraine and is there an aura that occurs before the onset of the headache?
2. Take a full gynaecological, obstetric, medical and surgical history along with medication, social and family history.
3. If migraine with aura is identified, combined hormonal contraception (CHC) is contraindicated, but all other methods could be offered. Explain why CHC is contraindicated – associated with an increased risk of stroke in women with migraine with aura.
4. Discuss the most suitable methods (progestogen-only methods, barrier methods and intrauterine devices).
5. Discussion includes mechanism of action, benefits, risks and side-effects, efficacy and time until the method becomes effective.
6. If the selected method is not immediately available, suggest a bridging method and arrange referral/appointment to have the method fitted, as appropriate.

2.5 Closing the session

- This provides an opportunity to summarize the session briefly and clarify the final choice of method of contraception.
- Routine follow-up is often not required; however, it is important that women feel they are able to re-attend if they have concerns or queries.
- Safety-nets should be established, with information provided about when to seek help and how to access support if there are any queries or concerns when the clinic or surgery is closed.

2.6 Summary

The contraception consultation is a rewarding and challenging undertaking. It incorporates clinician and patient agendas and, ideally, both are addressed resulting in a satisfactory outcome. The provision of accurate, up-to-date and applicable information empowers women to choose the method they would like. This increases the chance of ongoing and correct use, not to mention patient satisfaction.

References

FSRH (2017) *Quick Starting Contraception. Clinical effectiveness unit.* [www.fsrh.org/standards-and-guidance/documents/fsrh-clinical-guidance-quick-starting-contraception-april-2017 – accessed May 2023]

Home Office (2015, updated 2017) *FGM: mandatory reporting in healthcare.* [www.gov.uk/government/publications/fgm-mandatory-reporting-in-healthcare – accessed May 2023]

Kurtz, S., Silverman, J. and Draper, J. (2005) *Teaching and Learning Communication Skills in Medicine*, 2nd edition. CRC Press.

UKMEC (2016) *UK Medical Eligibility Criteria for Contraceptive Use* [www.fsrh.org/ukmec – accessed May 2023]

Chapter 3
Special groups

There are several groups for whom the provision of contraception can present additional challenges. This chapter considers these challenges in more detail and explores contraceptive provision for young people, those who identify as transgender or non-binary, those over 40 years, individuals with physical disabilities or learning difficulties, women living with HIV, and women with inflammatory bowel disease (IBD), cardiovascular disease, eating disorders and weight concerns, and those who are taking medications which may interact with contraception or have a teratogenic effect.

3.1 Young people

'Young people' refers to individuals under the age of 18 years. For those over 16 years an ability to consent is assumed unless there are additional factors such as a learning disability, which may affect an individual's ability to consent. For those under 16 years an assessment of competence to consent is undertaken at each attendance.

3.1.1 Consent

For an individual to be deemed able to consent they would be expected to demonstrate an ability to understand, retain and weigh up the information given to them regarding the intervention and then communicate their decision. Fraser guidelines provide a useful outline for this process (see *Box 3.1*); they are applicable to England, Wales and Northern Ireland. In Scotland the criteria which need to be met are that the individual understands the nature of the treatment offered and the consequences of that treatment.

At the beginning of the consultation there should be a discussion regarding the need to breach confidentiality if concerns arise. If concerns do arise, clinicians will take further action as necessary, in line with local policies and procedures.

3.1.2 Other issues

- For all consultations involving young and/or vulnerable individuals an assessment of potential abuse or exploitation is recommended.

Box 3.1. Fraser guidelines

- The young person understands the professional's advice.
- The young person cannot be persuaded to inform their parents.
- The young person is likely to begin or to continue having sex with or without contraceptive treatment.

- Unless the young person receives contraceptive treatment, their physical and/or mental health is likely to suffer.
- The young person's best interests require them to receive contraceptive advice or treatment with or without parental consent.

- Age is not a limiting factor to contraceptive choice, and a comprehensive history and discussion of available options enables young people to make an informed choice.
- During an ideal consultation sexual health, delaying sexual debut, legal issues, unintended pregnancy, condom use and STIs, including offering testing, are explored and discussed.
- Research suggests that the contraceptive choices made by young people are influenced by multiple factors including efficacy, safety, side-effect profile, invasiveness, ease of use and their knowledge of the method.
- In addition, young people often have particular areas of concern, for example, weight gain or acne, which if elicited and discussed may improve the acceptability of, and compliance with, a chosen method.

3.2 Women over 40 years of age

- Age alone is not a contraindication to the use of any method of contraception. The final decision is often based on the interplay between medical conditions, menstrual history and the acceptability of a method to a given individual.
- Over the age of 40 there is an age-related increased risk of cardiovascular disease, obesity and breast, endometrial and ovarian cancer which may affect contraceptive options.
  - A discussion of STI screening and symptoms is as important for women over 40 as it is for women of any other age group.
  - Eliciting any urogenital symptoms, sexual function concerns including libido, vaginal dryness and dyspareunia should ideally be included in the consultation.
- The average age of the menopause is 51–52 years. Women using non-hormonal contraceptives can be advised to stop their contraceptive after 1 year of amenorrhoea if they are over 50 years of age and after 2 years if under 50 years.
- The timing or duration of menopause is not affected by the use of contraception; however, use may mask menopausal symptoms.
- Women can stop contraception at the age of 55 as it is exceptionally rare for spontaneous conception to occur after this age.
- If women over the age of 50, using progestogen-only methods, wish to stop their contraception before the age of 55, an FSH level can be undertaken. If the FSH level is >30 IU/L, contraception can be discontinued in 12 months' time.
- POP and IMP are not associated with an increased risk of VTE, MI or stroke and have not been shown to affect BMD. There is no age restriction to the use of these methods.
- Peri-menopausal women taking CHCs may develop flushes and sweats in the hormone-free interval (HFI). Reducing the HFI to 4 days or using an extended regimen may alleviate these symptoms.
- For women over the age of 40, the lowest possible dose of oestrogen (<30 micrograms of ethinylestradiol or an oestradiol-containing CHC) along with levonorgestrel or norethisterone is recommended due to the lower risk of VTE, cardiovascular disease and stroke when compared with higher doses of oestrogen and the lower VTE risk associated with the aforementioned progestogens.

Furthermore, at the age of 50 years a CHC is normally changed to a progestogen-only method as the risks associated with CHC use outweigh the benefits.

- For those women using a progestogen-only injectable, it is advisable to consider an alternative method by the age of 50 years. However, if a woman wishes to continue to use this method, consideration regarding continuation should be based on the risks and benefits for a given individual and the decision should be regularly reviewed.
- Any copper intrauterine device inserted after the age of 40 can be used until contraception is no longer required, or 1 year after the menopause in the over 50s.
- A levonorgestrel intrauterine system (Mirena, containing 52 mg) fitted for contraception after the age of 45 can remain in place until a woman is 55. Removal after this time is recommended as there is a potential risk that the IUC may become a focus of infection.
- HRT is not a contraceptive. Progestogen-only methods and IUCs can be used alongside HRT.

3.3 Women living with HIV

- The British Association for Sexual Health and HIV and the British HIV Association have guidelines which include the use of contraception for women living with HIV.
- Prevention of transmission of HIV and other STIs is routinely discussed with women living with HIV, and safe sex promoted.
- Consistent condom use along with an additional contraceptive method (known as dual protection) is recommended for women living with HIV to prevent pregnancy and reduce horizontal transmission. Consistent use of a condom at each occurrence of sex in serodiscordant couples reduces the risk of HIV transmission by 80%. Condoms lubricated with the spermicide nonoxynol-9 (the only spermicide available in the UK) are not recommended because the spermicide can cause mucosal irritation and has been shown to increase the risk of HIV transmission.
- All methods of contraception are suitable for women who are not on antiretroviral therapy (ART).
- A discussion of all contraceptive methods with an explanation of potential drug interactions is recommended for women who are taking ART. If ART is a barrier to optimizing contraception because of drug interactions and alternative ART is available, a discussion with clinicians providing HIV care may be recommended to consider a change in ART.
- HIV drug interaction websites such as www.hiv-druginteractions.org provide a valuable reference for assessing potential drug interactions prior to commencing contraception.
- Many of the drugs which form part of ART interact with combined oral contraceptives, progestogen-only pills and contraceptive implants.
- The efficacy of the injectable contraceptive, IUSs and IUDs is not affected by ART.
- Due to a potentially higher risk of post-procedure infection, the initiation of IUCs is not recommended (UKMEC 3) for women living with HIV who have a CD4 count of <200 cells/mm^3.

- HIV infection appears to be associated with reduced bone density and individuals with HIV more commonly have osteopenia than the general population. In addition, the initiation of ART is associated with a loss in BMD before it stabilizes. Therefore a discussion of the risks and benefits of the progestogen-only injectable is advised, with re-evaluation every 2 years. NICE recommends vitamin D supplementation for those at increased risk of osteopenia or osteoporosis.
- Contraception method choice should not be restricted for women identified as being at high risk of HIV. All methods are UKMEC 1 for this group. This change to practice follows a WHO review of evidence including a high quality randomized control trial of IUD, IMP and progestogen-only injectable contraceptive use in women at high risk of HIV acquisition. The ECHO trial found no significant difference in HIV acquisition between the different methods.
- For those seeking emergency contraception a copper intrauterine device is first line. If an oral method is preferred, doubling the dose of levonorgestrel (3 mg) is recommended for women taking ART.
- Neither PEP nor PrEP are routinely recommended for the partners of women living with HIV if they are taking ART with a confirmed and sustained (>6 months) undetectable plasma HIV viral load (<200 copies/ml). Furthermore, following insertive vaginal intercourse with an HIV-positive partner not on ART, PEP should be 'considered' rather than routinely 'recommended' unless additional factors, such as high viral load, STIs or breaches in mucosal barrier, are present.
- The current recommendation for PrEP is to offer a daily oral tenofovir/emtricitabine (TD-FTC) to HIV-negative heterosexual men and women having condomless sex with partners who are HIV positive, unless the partner has been on ART for at least 6 months and their plasma viral load is <200 copies/ml.

3.4 Women with inflammatory bowel disease (IBD)

IBD, including ulcerative colitis and Crohn's disease, can present at any age, though it frequently presents between the ages of 10 and 40 years.

- When determining contraceptive options for a woman with IBD, a number of additional factors need to be considered:
  - the impact of the IBD on an individual's digestive tract and an individual's surgical history
  - the impact of IBD-associated conditions such as VTE, osteoporosis and hepatobiliary disease
  - the medications used in IBD management such as corticosteroids, immunosuppressants, 5-aminosalicylic acid drugs and anti-tumour necrosis factor alpha agents, which aim to reduce and prevent recurrence.
- A causal relationship between COC use and the onset or exacerbation of IBD has not been established.
- The efficacy of oral contraceptives is unlikely to be reduced in women with large bowel disease. However, it may be reduced in women with small bowel disease and malabsorption.

- There is no evidence to suggest IBD reduces the efficacy of the CTP, IMP, progestogen-only injectable or IUC.
- Rectal preparations for IBD, such as oil- or Witepsol-based products, may reduce the efficacy of latex barrier methods if the product spreads to genital skin, therefore a review of the constituents of products used is advisable for those using these barrier methods.
- Previous pelvic or abdominal surgery may affect the safety and success of laparoscopic sterilization. In these circumstances a LARC or vasectomy are good alternatives.
- Crohn's & Colitis UK produce a useful information sheet on reproductive health and IBD, available at: https://s3-eu-west-1.amazonaws.com/files.crohnsandcolitis.org.uk/Publications/Reproductive_Health.pdf.

3.4.1 Pregnancy and IBD

- Encourage women to plan to conceive when their disease is controlled.
- Contraception enables women to optimize their IBD management. Pre-pregnancy counselling may be available locally depending on provision.
- The impact of all medications on pregnancy should be reviewed with women and men with IBD who are considering pregnancy.
- Crohn's & Colitis UK produce a helpful information sheet on pregnancy and IBD, available at: https://s3-eu-west-1.amazonaws.com/files.crohnsandcolitis.org.uk/Publications/Pregnancy_and_IBD.

3.5 Women with cardiovascular disease

- For young women with cardiovascular disease, the provision of contraception and sexual health advice should ideally occur as part of transitional care from paediatric to adult services. Discussions should cover the significance of an individual's cardiac disease in terms of risk associated with pregnancy, risk of thrombosis, severe vasovagal reaction and endocarditis, contraception (if any methods are contraindicated), sexual activity and sexual function.
- Involving the young woman and all members of the healthcare team, including the individual's cardiologist, ensures both medical and personal acceptability of the contraceptive method.
- CHCs are associated with an increased risk of VTE and are often contraindicated in women with cardiovascular disease.
- Prophylactic antibiotics are not required for the insertion of IUCs in women at risk of infective endocarditis. More complex individual cases, such as those with a past history of endocarditis, structural congenital heart disease or prosthetic heart valve, should be discussed with a cardiologist.
- For women at increased risk of vasovagal reactions, or those with a complex cardiac history in whom a vasovagal episode could present a very high risk, discussion with cardiology is advised and insertion of an IUC should occur in a hospital setting, with appropriate resuscitation support available.

- The use of anticoagulant therapy (warfarin, low molecular weight heparin and direct anticoagulants) need not restrict the provision of IMP or IUCs, providing there are no additional factors in an individual's history which may indicate a higher risk of bleeding. For women with an increased risk of bleeding, for example an INR >3.5, discussion of their case with haematology and arranging for insertion to occur in a hospital setting may be considered. In general anticoagulants should not be stopped prior to contraception-related procedures, as the risk of clot formation outweighs the small risk of bleeding.
- A desogestrel-containing progestogen-only contraceptive pill is a useful interim method (except for women using liver enzyme inducers) to prevent pregnancy while obtaining further information and clarification from the woman's cardiologist.

3.6 Weight concerns – obesity, weight reduction medication/surgery, weight gain and contraception

- When compared to women with a normal BMI (<25 kg/m^2), those with obesity (BMI >30 kg/m^2) have an increased risk of conditions including VTE, hypertension, type 2 diabetes, breast and endometrial cancer. In addition, women with obesity who become pregnant are at risk of pregnancy-related complications including hypertension, diabetes, pre-eclampsia, post-partum haemorrhage, fetal growth restriction, macrosomia, neural tube defects and stillbirth.
- Consideration of the use of weight-loss medication, both on prescription and over the counter, as well as laxatives is important, as this may influence contraceptive method choice.
- The contraception consultation may provide an opportunity to sensitively discuss weight in the context of contraception and fertility and signpost to support available if desired.
- The IUC, IMP and POP are safe and effective methods for women who have a BMI >25 kg/m^2. There is no need to alter duration of use or dosage. The IMP should not be more difficult to remove in women with a raised BMI, providing it was initially inserted correctly.
- Oral EC, particularly LNG-EC, may be less effective in women weighing >70 kg or with a BMI >26 kg/m^2. If a Cu-IUD is not indicated or not acceptable, UPA-EC can be offered. If UPA-EC is not suitable, a double dose (3 mg) of LNG-EC can be used.
- The progestogen-only injectable contraceptive is effective for women with a BMI >25 kg/m^2. While obesity does not restrict the use of this method, if a raised BMI is one of multiple risk factors for cardiovascular disease (other risk factors include smoking, diabetes and hypertension), an alternative method is recommended. For women wishing to use this method it may be more practical to use a longer needle or inject into the deltoid, or change to the subcutaneous preparation Sayana Press.
- The risks generally outweigh the benefits for COC use in women with a BMI >35 kg/m^2 and for those with a BMI of between 30 and 34 kg/m^2 who have other risk factors for cardiovascular disease. In women with a BMI >25 kg/m^2 there

may be increased ovarian activity in the HFI compared to women with a normal BMI; therefore tailored use of the COC may be the most effective way to use this method. The CTP may be less effective for women weighing more than 90 kg.

- There are no known drug interactions between medications for weight loss (orlistat, liraglutide and naltrexone/bupropion) and hormonal contraception. However, diarrhoea can be induced by these medications, which may reduce the absorption and potentially decrease the effectiveness of oral contraception.
- Women who have had bariatric surgery should avoid pregnancy for 12–18 months post procedure and during times of significant active weight loss. IUC and IMP are thought to be safe and effective for use following bariatric surgery. The absorption and efficacy of oral contraception may be reduced as a result of surgery, therefore alternative methods are recommended. Both the progestogen-only injectable and bariatric surgery are associated with a reduction in bone mineral density which should be discussed as alternative methods may be preferable.
- Although some women do gain weight while using contraception, there is no evidence that the use of intrauterine contraception, IMP, POP or CHC causes significant weight gain.
- Evidence of a relationship between progestogen-only injectable contraception and weight is variable. Its use appears to be associated with some weight gain, particularly in women aged under 18 with a BMI ≥30 kg/m². Women who gain more than 5% of their baseline body weight in the first 6 months of use may be more likely to experience continued weight gain. However, data is insufficient to confirm or exclude a causal relationship between progestogen-only injectable use and weight gain.
- The perception that weight gain is a side-effect of contraceptive use is often cited by women as a reason not to initiate or to discontinue their contraception. Clear explanation that there is no evidence to support this, and that women tend to gain weight over time regardless of the use of contraception, may reduce discontinuation rates.

3.7 Women with eating disorders

- Eating disorders include anorexia nervosa, bulimia nervosa, binge eating disorder and other specified feeding or eating disorder (OSFED). Abnormal attitudes and behaviour towards eating and distorted body self-image characterize these disorders.
- Even though menstrual irregularities, amenorrhoea and anovulation are common, effective contraception is required by sexually active women of reproductive age with eating disorders. It is important that the risk of pregnancy, despite the presence of menstrual irregularities, is clearly explained in order to facilitate a discussion of contraceptive options.
- In addition, due to the increased risk of adverse pregnancy outcomes (including hyperemesis, anaemia, intrauterine growth restriction and preterm birth) associated with being underweight at the time of conception, delaying pregnancy until a woman's eating disorder is in remission is recommended.

- When deliberating contraceptive options there are several additional factors to consider and discuss:
  - Consideration of laxative use and the practice of self-induced vomiting is important. There is very limited evidence on the effect of laxative misuse on the efficacy of oral contraceptives. However, the absorption of oral contraceptives may be affected indirectly by drugs that cause vomiting or severe diarrhoea, or by drugs that alter gut transit. In the presence of such practices the use of non-oral methods or LARCs may be more advantageous.
  - Women with eating disorders and very little subcutaneous tissue may be at increased risk of deep implant insertion. In addition, the implant may be more visible in very thin arms.
  - For those who select IUC, a smaller than typical device may be required due to an atrophic and small uterus. In addition, anorexia is associated with an increased risk of the development of cardiac abnormalities, including bradycardia, low blood pressure and prolonged QT interval (UKMEC 3). Furthermore, a pre-existing slow pulse and/or low blood pressure may increase the chance of a vasovagal episode occurring during or after IUC fitting; equally, there is a risk of a vasovagal episode occurring at the time of insertion of an IUC in women who have not eaten on the day of fitting.
  - While there is no evidence that hormonal contraception causes weight gain (with the exception of DMPA; see *Section 3.6*), body changes such as breast enlargement and bloating can be associated with hormonal contraception, and these changes may cause additional distress.
  - Osteoporosis and osteopenia are common in women with anorexia and a significantly lower BMD is seen in women with bulimia when compared to healthy controls. The reason for this alteration in BMD is thought to be multifactorial, not solely due to weight loss. Although it is common practice to use CHC to provide bone protection, evidence demonstrates that CHC is not effective in increasing BMD in women with anorexia. While there is no evidence of the effect of DMPA on the BMD of women with eating disorders, it is known that DMPA is associated with a small reduction in BMD during use, which is largely recoverable on cessation. In view of this, prior to commencing or continuing DMPA in women with eating disorders an informed discussion and consideration of alternatives is recommended.

3.8 Drug interactions

- Prior to the provision of contraception it is important to ask about current medication, including over-the-counter and herbal remedies to ascertain if they interact with an individual's chosen method.
- Likewise, before new medication is commenced women are advised to discuss their current contraception use in order to avoid potential drug interactions.
- Liver enzyme inducing drugs reduce the bioavailability of oestrogen and progestogen and so potentially reduce the contraceptive efficacy of several methods of contraception.

- Progestogen-only injectables, IUS and IUD are unaffected by liver enzyme inducing drugs.
- It is advisable for women to use additional barrier methods or change to an injectable or IUC when liver enzyme inducing medications are commenced (see *Table 3.1* for common liver enzyme inducing drugs).
- Some women will only use enzyme inducing medications on a short-term basis and may wish to remain on their current CHC, POP or IMP. The addition of a barrier method for the duration of the treatment and for 28 days after stopping the drug is recommended as an alternative to a change in method.
  - If a CHC is to be continued, prescribe a COC containing a minimum of 30 micrograms ethinylestradiol or a patch or vaginal ring. Advocate an extended cycle regimen or tricycling (taking 3 packets back to back) and reduce the HFI to 4 days PLUS use a barrier method.
  - Alternatively, increase ethinylestradiol to at least 50 micrograms (taking a 20 and 30 micrograms COC) using the extended cycle regimen or tricycling with a 4 day HFI. Using two vaginal rings or two patches is not recommended. This approach is not advised for those taking rifampicin or rifabutin. Women using these medications should always be advised to change to an alternative method.
- If emergency contraception is required, a copper IUD is first line due to the potential interaction between oral emergency contraception and liver enzyme inducing drugs. If an IUD is declined or unsuitable a 3 mg dose (double dose) of oral levonorgestrel as soon as possible within 120 hours of unprotected sex can be used. This use is outside the product licence.
- Ulipristal acetate (emergency contraception) is not advised for women currently using, or who have used enzyme inducing drugs in the last 28 days.
- There is no need to use additional contraception during or after a course of non-enzyme inducing antibiotics.
- CHC and lamotrigine monotherapy are not recommended due to the risk of reduced seizure control whilst on CHC and potential toxicity during the CHC-free interval. The POP may increase lamotrigine levels, therefore monitoring for side-effects is recommended if this method is to be used. There is a possible risk that

Table 3.1 Liver enzyme inducing drugs

Drug category	Medication		
Antibiotic	Rifabutin Rifampicin		
Antiepileptic	Carbamazepine Eslicarbazepine Phenytoin	Primidone Rifinamide Topiramate	Lamotrigine
Antiretroviral	See HIV Drug Interaction Checker (www.hiv-druginteractions.org)		
Herbal	St John's wort		
Other	Aprepitant Bosentan Sugammadex		

lamotrigine may affect POP and implant efficacy so, 'erring on the side of caution', FSRH CEU suggest additional condom use. All other methods are suitable.

- In those taking thyroxine it is possible that the dose may need to be increased when a CHC is started, due to the effect of oestrogen on thyroid-binding globulin levels.
- Useful sources to review interactions are the *British National Formulary* (*BNF*) and *Stockley's Drug Interactions* (www.medicinescomplete.com/mc/index.htm).

3.9 Teratogenic drugs or drugs with potential teratogenic effects

- Teratogenic medications are known to have, or are suspected of having the potential to increase the risk of birth defects and developmental disorders in pregnancy, especially during the first trimester.
- The UK Teratology Information Service (UKTIS) website (www.uktis.org) provides useful information regarding these medications.
- Women of reproductive age, who are taking known teratogenic drugs or drugs with potential teratogenic effects, or are the partners of those taking known teratogenic drugs, should be made aware of the risks associated with these medications. Furthermore they should be advised to avoid unintended pregnancy by using highly effective contraception during treatment and for the recommended timeframe after discontinuation.
- The methods of contraception which are considered to be highly effective (<1% failure rate) are the LARCs: IUD, IUS and IMP, as well as male and female sterilization. Additional contraceptive precautions (e.g. condoms or a second effective contraceptive method) are not required if these methods are being used.
- Given the typical failure rates of CHC and POP (9%) and DMPA (6%) and the importance of avoiding pregnancy, it is recommended that users of these methods use additional contraceptive precautions, e.g. condoms.
- The sole use of barrier methods, withdrawal and fertility awareness is not recommended.
- It is very important to consider any other medication, e.g. liver enzyme inducing medication, which may potentially reduce the efficacy of a chosen method of contraception (see *Section 3.8*).
- Assessment for the likelihood of pregnancy should occur before each prescription of teratogenic medication, together with review of the method of contraception used and the reliability and consistency of that use. Depending on this risk assessment, pregnancy testing may be recommended. It may be advisable to provide a prescription of a shorter duration to women who use contraceptive methods that require frequent pregnancy testing. The Medicines for Women's Health Expert Advisory Group has created an aide memoire summary table to assist in this decision-making process, available at: https://assets.publishing.service.gov.uk/media/5c936a4840f0b633f5bfd895/pregnancy_testing_and_contraception_table_for_medicines_with_teratogenic_potential_final.pdf.

- All oral retinoids have an associated Pregnancy Prevention Programme, which is supported by educational material for prescribers, pharmacists and patients: www. gov.uk/drug-safety-update/oral-retinoids-pregnancy-prevention-reminder-of-measures-to-minimise-teratogenic-risk.
- The valproate pregnancy prevention programme has been in place since April 2018 when the licence for prescribing valproate changed; it aims to minimize the potential risks of valproate during pregnancy. Valproate should only be prescribed to women of child-bearing age when there are no alternative treatments and the conditions of the pregnancy prevention programme have been met, irrespective of the indication for the prescription. As part of this programme, health professionals have specific responsibilities including:
  - GPs: recall all women and girls who may have child-bearing potential, provide the Patient Guide, check they have been reviewed by a specialist in the last year, have an in-date Risk Acknowledgement Form and are on highly effective contraception
  - specialists: review women at least annually to re-evaluate treatment as necessary, explain clearly the conditions as outlined in the supporting materials and complete and sign the Annual Risk Acknowledgement Form with copies for the patient or carer and the GP
  - pharmacists: dispense whole packs of medication whenever possible; packs should have a warning label either on the carton or via a sticker. At the time of dispensing, the risk of pregnancy and contraception use should be discussed, patient guides (leaflet and card) provided and date since last review with GP or specialist to discuss treatment and complete the Risk Acknowledgement Form determined.

3.10 Transgender and non-binary individuals

- A transgender individual is someone whose gender identity does not correlate exactly with the sex assigned to them at birth.
- Non-binary describes a gender identity which is not exclusively binary male or female.
- A cisgender individual is someone whose gender identity correlates with the sex assigned to them at birth.
- Sensitive, individualized discussion, ascertaining the need for contraception and sexual health care, is an important component of providing medical care to all individuals.
- The requirement for hormonal and/or surgical treatment and the acceptability of specific methods of contraception is highly individual.
- There is limited research evidence pertaining to contraception options, particularly with regard to effectiveness and safety, for transgender and non-binary individuals. Therefore, advice is based on expert opinion.
- Transgender and non-binary individuals should be offered all the forms of contraception offered to cisgender individuals. There are no restrictions to the use of any method of contraception for people assigned female at birth because of their current gender identity.

- As with cisgender individuals, medical, family and drug history are the key determinants of medical eligibility for the various methods of contraception (see *Chapter 2*). This is then followed by the provision of information about available methods to enable decision-making.
- Cervical and breast screening are recommended for individuals with a cervix and those with any breast tissue (in addition, breast screening is recommended for transwomen using hormonal therapy which increases the risk of breast cancer). Invitations for screening are based on whether an individual is registered with their general practitioner as male or female. Invitations can be obtained via GP referral to the screening programme as needed. For more information see Public Health England or Wales screening programmes.
- Individuals using testosterone therapy or gonadotrophin-releasing hormone analogues to suppress ovarian function should be aware that neither provide contraception; the presence of amenorrhoea does not mean there is not risk of pregnancy. Furthermore, testosterone is potentially teratogenic, therefore pregnancy is an absolute contraindication to testosterone therapy.
- There are no contraindications to the concomitant use of testosterone with any method of contraception; the choice of methods should be determined by the individual requiring contraception and their preference, depending on medical eligibility.
- There may be a preference for a method where the route of delivery is desexualized. An individual may experience pelvic dysphoria or have hypo-oestrogenized vaginal tissue, or may benefit from a very detailed description of the steps undertaken when an IUD is inserted.
- Sexual health advice, including condom use and STIs, vaccination and discussion of PEP and PrEP, is recommended, with additional information provided as required.

3.11 Women with learning disabilities

- Learning disabilities are a spectrum of disorders wherein an individual has a reduced ability to understand new or complex information and may be unable to live independently.
- Women with learning disabilities should be supported to make their own decisions about contraception. Studies have shown that individuals with learning disabilities have a lower knowledge base about contraceptive methods than women without disabilities. Therefore provision of accessible information is an important part of the decision-making process. A person with a learning disability may still be competent to make an informed choice regarding a method of contraception and be able to use any method reliably, including an oral method. Discussion of available options is based on medical assessment and the acceptability of a method to a given individual, not their learning disability.

3.11.1 Consent and capacity

- To be deemed competent an individual must demonstrate an ability to understand and retain the information provided, weigh up the risks and benefits and express their wishes as set out in the Mental Capacity Act 2005 for England and Wales. The Act applies to all individuals aged 16 years and over. Under the Act a person is presumed to be competent unless they have demonstrated otherwise. Competence is decision-specific and cannot be generalized to all medical situations.

- When a woman with a learning disability is unable to understand and take responsibility for her decisions about contraception, a meeting between carers and other involved parties is advised. This discussion aims to establish a care plan, address issues around the woman's contraceptive need but also consider the individual's wishes too. Any decision made is in the best interests of the individual and generally the least restrictive option. No one individual can consent for another.

- If a woman has no-one (other than paid carers) to support and represent her, or when a serious medical treatment such as sterilization or abortion is proposed, an Independent Mental Capacity Advocate (IMCA) is appointed. Their role is to support an individual to ensure that they can participate in decision making, to determine their wishes, beliefs and values, and to discuss alternative options. Those involved in the care of an individual with an IMCA are obliged to take into consideration submissions made by the IMCA.

- When making decisions regarding contraception for an individual with learning disabilities the best interests of that person are paramount rather than opting for the most convenient option for those involved in supporting/caring for that individual. Importantly, carers cannot give consent for another individual.

- The Court of Protection was established under the Mental Capacity Act and its role is to protect those who lack capacity and make rulings on difficult decisions regarding their care. An application may be made to the Court of Protection by a family member, hospital trust or local authority. The decision making process involves the individual who lacks capacity. A 'litigation friend' is appointed to provide legal instruction; this may be a friend, relative or solicitor. If no-one is available, an official solicitor is appointed to act as a litigation friend during the Court of Protection process.

3.12 Women with physical disabilities

Women with physical disabilities requiring contraception should be supported in making their own decisions.

- It is important to consider the impact of a physical disability on an individual's mobility when discussing contraceptive options.

- For women with very limited mobility it is wise to review their baseline risk of VTE and the impact of the additional risk associated with oestrogen-containing methods of contraception before prescribing.

- For women with limited mobility or those with a medical condition which may affect bone mineral density, careful consideration of the risks and benefits is advisable before prescribing progestogen-only injectable contraceptives (see *Section 6.6*).

- For those with limited dexterity, for example, due to arthritis, consideration should be given to the administration of contraceptive methods to ensure that their disability does not unduly limit their choice of contraception. Dexterity may limit the ability of an individual to utilize oral contraceptives or patches or vaginal rings.

3.13 Women with sensory disabilities

3.13.1 Visual impairment

- Research indicates that young adults with visual impairments have similar rates of sexual experiences as their sighted counterparts; however, their experience typically occurs 2–3 years later, highlighting the importance of considering their sexual health needs.
- The provision of information in large print, Braille or as a recording is important for clients with visual impairments.
- There should be access to advocates for women with sensory impairments.
- For visually impaired women wishing to use a COC or a POP, the pharmacy or family members may need to include the contraceptive in a 'dosette box'. This will help compliance and ensure this method of contraception is an option for visually impaired women because Braille packaging is not generally available.

3.13.2 Hearing impairment

- Studies have shown that individuals with hearing impairment have a lower knowledge base about contraceptive methods than women without. Therefore provision of accessible information is hugely important to enable women to make their own decision regarding their choice of contraception.
- For women with hearing impairments who lip read, face to face consultation with slow, clear articulation, avoiding over-exaggerated facial expression, can be sufficient to ensure an effective consultation. Individuals with a strongly accented voice may find it more difficult to undertake the consultation because accents can make lip reading more difficult.
- There should be access to advocates for women with sensory impairments.
- The provision of an interpreter for deaf clients may be required, depending on clinician or client request, with care taken to ensure privacy but also to ensure the woman has a 'voice' during intimate examinations.

3.14 Women who do not speak English

- For clients who do not have English as a first language, the provision of an interpreter may be needed.
- The interpreter should not be a family member, but an independent individual who acts purely as a channel for communication. The interpreter may be physically present at the time of the consultation or participate via telephone.

- For intimate examinations, it is generally recommended that an interpreter is present within the consultation room.

EXAMPLE

A 24 year old woman with learning disabilities attends with her mum who is requesting a sterilization for her daughter.

What should you do?

1. Discuss the reasons behind the request.
2. Ascertain the young woman's wishes through an IMCA if necessary.
3. Consider less permanent options.
4. Refer to the Court of Protection if a decision cannot be reached.

References

BHIVA (2015) *UK Guideline for the Use of HIV Post-Exposure Prophylaxis Following Sexual Exposure (PEPSE).*
[www.bashh.org/documents/PEPSE%202015%20guideline%20final_NICE.pdf – accessed May 2023]

BHIVA/BASHH (2018) *Guidelines on the Use of HIV Pre-Exposure Prophylaxis (PrEP).*
[www.bhiva.org/file/5b729cd592060/2018-PrEP-Guidelines.pdf – accessed May 2023]

Boudreau, D. and Mukerjee, R. (2019) Contraception care for transmasculine individuals on testosterone therapy. *Journal of Midwifery and Women's Health*, **64(4)**: 395–402.
[https://onlinelibrary.wiley.com/doi/epdf/10.1111/jmwh.12962 – accessed May 2023]

Evidence for Contraceptive Options and HIV Outcomes (ECHO) Trial Consortium (2019) HIV incidence among women using intramuscular depot medroxyprogesterone acetate, a copper intrauterine device, or a levonorgestrel implant for contraception: a randomised, multicentre, open-label trial. *Lancet*, **394**: 303–13.
[www.thelancet.com/journals/lancet/article/PIIS0140-6736(19)31288-7/fulltext#%20 – accessed May 2023]

Fakoya, A. *et al.* (2008) *UK guidelines for the management of sexual and reproductive health (SRH) of people living with HIV infection.* BASHH and BHIVA.
[available at www.bashhguidelines.org/media/1068/sexual-reproductive-health.pdf – accessed May 2023]

FSRH (2010, amended 2019) *Contraceptive Choices for Young People.* Clinical Effectiveness Unit.
[www.fsrh.org/documents/cec-ceu-guidance-young-people-mar-2010/fsrh-guideline-contraception-young-people-may-2019.pdf – accessed May 2023]

FSRH (2014) *Contraceptive Choices for Women with Cardiac Disease.* Clinical Effectiveness Unit. [www.fsrh.org/documents/ceu-guidance-contraceptive-choices-for-women-with-cardiac/ – accessed May 2023]

FSRH (2016) *Sexual and Reproductive Health for Individuals with Inflammatory Bowel Disease.* Clinical Effectiveness Unit. [www.fsrh.org/standards-and-guidance/documents/ceu-clinical-guidance-srh-ibd – accessed May 2023]

FSRH (2017) *CEU Statement: contraceptive choices and sexual health for transgender and non-binary people.* [www.fsrh.org/standards-and-guidance/documents/fsrh-ceu-statement-contraceptive-choices-and-sexual-health-for – accessed May 2023]

FSRH (2017) *CEU Statement: management of women taking anticoagulants or antiplatelet medications who request intrauterine contraception or subdermal implants.* Clinical Effectiveness Unit. [www.fsrh.org/standards-and-guidance/documents/fsrh-guidance-fsrh-guidance-management-of-women-taking – accessed May 2023]

FSRH (2017, amended 2019) *Contraception for Women Aged Over 40.* Clinical Effectiveness Unit. [www.fsrh.org/standards-and-guidance/documents/fsrh-guidance-contraception-for-women-aged-over-40-years-2017 – accessed May 2023]

FSRH (2018, updated 2021) *CEU Statement: contraception for women with eating disorders.* Clinical Effectiveness Unit. [www.fsrh.org/standards-and-guidance/documents/fsrh-ceu-statement-contraception-for-women-with-eating – accessed May 2023]

FSRH (2018) *CEU Statement: contraception for women using known teratogenic drugs or drugs with potential teratogenic effects.* Clinical Effectiveness Unit. [www.fsrh.org/standards-and-guidance/documents/fsrh-ceu-statement-contraception-for-women-using-known – accessed May 2023]

FSRH (2019) *Overweight, Obesity & Contraception.* Clinical Effectiveness Unit. [www.fsrh.org/standards-and-guidance/documents/fsrh-clinical-guideline-overweight-obesity-and-contraception – accessed May 2023]

FSRH (2019) *CEU Statement: contraception and weight gain.* Clinical Effectiveness Unit. [www.fsrh.org/standards-and-guidance/documents/fsrh-ceu-statement-contraception-and-weight-gain-august-2019 – accessed May 2023]

FSRH (2022) *CEU Guidance: drug interactions with hormonal contraception.* Clinical Effectiveness Unit. [www.fsrh.org/standards-and-guidance/fsrh-guidelines-and-statements/drug-interactions – accessed May 2023]

Mental Capacity Act (2005)
[www.legislation.gov.uk/ukpga/2005/9/contents – accessed May 2023]

MHRA (2018, updated 2021) *Valproate Use by Women and Girls.*
[www.gov.uk/guidance/valproate-use-by-women-and-girls – accessed May 2023]

MHRA (2019) *Drug Safety Update* volume 12, issue 8: March 2019: 3
[www.gov.uk/drug-safety-update/medicines-with-teratogenic-potential-what-is-effective-contraception-and-how-often-is-pregnancy-testing-needed#download-print-and-use-new-table – accessed May 2023]

Public Health England (PHE) (2017) *Information for Trans People – NHS Screening Programmes.*
[https://phescreening.blog.gov.uk/2017/07/04/new-leaflet-aims-to-improve-accessibility-to-screening-for-transgender-people – accessed May 2023]

Public Health Wales (2019) *Screening Information for Transgender Service Users.*
[https://phw.nhs.wales/services-and-teams/screening – accessed May 2023]

Waters, L. *et al.* (2017) BHIVA/BASHH/FSRH *Guidelines for the Sexual and Reproductive Health of People living with HIV* (consultation document).
[www.bhiva.org/guidelines – accessed May 2023]

Chapter 4

Combined hormonal contraception

Approximately 3 million UK women use the combined oral contraceptive (COC).

Combined hormonal contraceptives (CHCs) contain both oestrogen and progestogen. There are three routes of administration: oral (pill), transdermal (combined transdermal patch, CTP) and vaginal (combined vaginal ring, CVR).

In addition to its contraceptive indication, CHCs are prescribed to help manage menstrual symptoms including dysmenorrhoea, premenstrual syndrome, heavy menstrual bleeding and acne. Only one product (Qlaira) has a licence for the treatment of heavy menstrual bleeding in those who desire contraception. Prescribing solely for a non-contraceptive benefit is seen as an off-licence indication.

4.1 Potential users

4.1.1 Most appropriate users

- CHCs can be used from menarche to the age of 50 years providing there are no contraindicating risk factors or medical conditions. For those over 50, healthcare professionals can use their clinical judgement; however, the risk generally outweighs the benefit.
- CHCs are an ideal choice for women who wish to have a regular bleed or to control when they have a withdrawal bleed.
- Individuals should choose whether they wish to use oral, transdermal or vaginal CHCs.

4.1.2 Not suitable for the following users

CHCs are not suitable for the following women:
- those who suffer from migraine with aura
- those with current or recent breast cancer
- those breastfeeding and less than 6 weeks post-partum
- those less than 3 weeks post-partum or less than 6 weeks post-partum with other risk factors for VTE, such as immobility, transfusion at delivery, BMI ≥30 kg/m², post-partum haemorrhage, post-caesarean delivery, pre-eclampsia or smoking
- those with a BMI over 35 kg/m²
- those with hypertension
- those over 35 years of age who currently smoke, including those who smoke electronic cigarettes, as the risk associated with electronic cigarette smoking has not yet been established
- those with multiple risk factors for arterial cardiovascular disease
- those with current or past VTE, or with VTE in a first-degree relative under the age of 45, or a known thrombogenic mutation
- those with known genetic mutation associated with breast cancer
- those with diabetes with retinopathy, nephropathy, neuropathy or other vascular disease

- those who have had bariatric surgery
- those experiencing prolonged immobility including following surgery
- those with acute or flare of viral hepatitis
- those with cirrhosis or liver tumours
- those with a current or history of ischaemic heart disease
- those with a current or history of stroke
- those with positive antiphospholipid antibodies.

4.2 Available CHC in the UK

CHCs available in the UK are detailed in *Table 4.1*, along with associated costs and formulations. First-line choices are those containing ≤30 micrograms of ethinylestradiol and either levonorgestrel and norethisterone (highlighted in bold in table). There are currently no low ethinylestradiol dose and norethisterone-containing products on the UK market.

Table 4.1 CHCs available in the UK

Type of preparation	Trade name	Oestrogen and progestogen	Cost for 3 cycles Drug tariff price (NHS indicative price)
Monophasic low strength	Bimizza Gedarel 20/150 Mercilon	Ethinylestradiol 20 micrograms Desogestrel 150 micrograms	£5.98 (£5.04) £5.98 (£5.04) £5.98 (£5.04)
	Akizza 20/75 Femodette Millinette 20/75 Sunya 20/75	Gestodene 75 micrograms	£8.85 (£6.73) £8.85 (£8.85) £8.85 (£6.37) £8.85 (£6.62)
Monophasic standard strength	Cimizt Gedarel 30/150 Marvelon	Desogestrel 150 micrograms	£4.93 (£3.80) £4.93 (£4.93) £4.93 (£7.10)
	Dretine Lucette Yacella Yasmin Yiznell	Ethinylestradiol 30 micrograms Drospirenone 3 mg	£14.70 (£8.34) £14.70 (£11.00) £14.70 (£8.30) £14.70 (£14.70) £14.70 (£8.30)
	Akizza 30/75 Femodene Katya 30/75 Millinette 30/75	Gestodene 75 micrograms	£8.85 (£6.73) £6.73 (£6.73) £6.73 (£5.03) £6.73 (£4.85)

(continued)

Type of preparation	Trade name	Oestrogen and progestogen			Cost for 3 cycles Drug tariff price (NHS indicative price)	
Monophasic standard strength (*cont'd*)	Ambelina Elevin Levest Maexeni Microgynon 30 Ovranette Rigevidon	Ethinylestradiol 30 micrograms			£2.82 (£2.60) £2.82 (£29.25) £2.82 (£1.80) £2.82 (£1.88) £2.82 (£2.82) £2.82 (£2.20) £2.82 (£1.89)	
Alternative monophasic options	Cilique Lizinna	Ethinylestradiol 35 micrograms Norgestimate 250 micrograms			£4.65 (£4.65) £4.65 (£4.64)	
	Brevinor	Ethinylestradiol 35 micrograms Norethisterone 500 micrograms			£1.99 (£1.99)	
	Norimin	Ethinylestradiol 35 micrograms Norethisterone 1 mg			£2.28 (£2.28)	
	Norinyl-1	Mestranol 50 micrograms Norethisterone 1 mg			£2.19 (£2.19)	
Monophasic 28-day preparations	Drovelis	Estetrol 14.2 mg Drospirenone 3 mg			Not available (£8.60)	
	Eloine	Ethinylestradiol 20 micrograms Drospirenone 3 mg			£14.70 (£14.70)	
	Femodene ED	Ethinylestradiol 30 micrograms Gestodene 75 micrograms			£7.10	
	Microgynon 30 ED	Ethinylestradiol 30 micrograms Levonorgestrel 150 micrograms			£2.99	
	Zoely	Oestradiol (as hemihydrate) 1.5 mg Nomegestrol acetate 2.5 mg			£19.80 (£19.80)	
Phasic standard strength	Logynon TriRegol	Ethinylestradiol 30 micrograms Ethinylestradiol 30 micrograms Ethinylestradiol 30 micrograms	Levonorgestrel 50 micrograms Levonorgestrel 75 micrograms Levonorgestrel 125 micrograms	6 5 10	£3.83 £2.43	
	Synphase	Ethinylestradiol 35 micrograms Ethinylestradiol 35 micrograms Ethinylestradiol 35 micrograms	Norethisterone 500 micrograms Norethisterone 1mg Norethisterone 500 micrograms	7 9 5	£3.60	
Phasic standard strength every day	Logynon ED	Ethinylestradiol 30 micrograms Ethinylestradiol 30 micrograms Ethinylestradiol 30 micrograms	Levonorgestrel 50 micrograms Levonorgestrel 75 micrograms Levonorgestrel 125 micrograms	6 5 10	£4.00	

Type of preparation	Trade name	Oestrogen and progestogen		Cost for 3 cycles Drug tariff price (NHS indicative price)
Phasic every day, 26 active and 2 inactive	Qlaira	Oestradiol valerate 3 mg	Dienogest 2 mg	2 £25.18
		Oestradiol valerate 2 mg	Dienogest 2 mg	5
		Oestradiol valerate 2 mg	Dienogest 3 mg	17
		Oestradiol valerate 1 mg	Dienogest 3 mg	2
Patch	Evra	Ethinylestradiol approx. 33.9 micrograms/ 24 hours Norelgestromin approx. 203 micrograms/24 hours		£19.51 (£19.51)
Ring	NuvaRing SyreniRing	Ethinylestradiol approx. 15 micrograms/24 hours Etonogestrel approx. 120 micrograms/24 hours		£29.70 (£29.70) £29.70 (£19.00)

Data from *BNF*, 2023.

4.3 Mechanism of action

- The main mode of action is the prevention of ovulation through negative feedback on the pituitary gland, inhibiting the release of luteinizing hormone (LH) and follicle-stimulating hormone (FSH). In formulations with 21 days of active hormone, the first 7 days of CHC use results in ovulation inhibition and the next 14 days maintains anovulation.
- Cervical mucus is altered which inhibits penetration of spermatozoa.
- Endometrial growth is suppressed, reducing the likelihood of blastocyst implantation.

4.4 Efficacy of CHC

If used consistently and correctly the failure rate for CHC is 0.3% (in the first year of use 3 in 1000 women would become pregnant) but this increases to 9% with typical use. The efficacy of CHC is affected by drug interactions, and the efficacy of the CTP may be reduced in women weighing >90 kg. LARCs are more effective than CHCs.

4.5 Pros and cons of CHC

4.5.1 Advantages

- Effective, reversible, convenient.
- Under user's control and unrelated to sexual intercourse.
- Provides regular, predictable withdrawal bleeds.
- Reduces menstrual loss by at least 40% – recommended by NICE (NG88, 2018) for the treatment of heavy menstrual bleeding.

- Decreases dysmenorrhoea and relieves ovulation pain.
- Reduces acne.
- May improve premenstrual symptoms.
- Protects against ectopic pregnancy because it inhibits ovulation.
- Reduces incidence of benign breast disease.
- Reduces the risk of ovarian cancer. A recent meta-analysis determined a significant duration–response relationship, with a reduction in the incidence of ovarian cancer of more than 50% among women using the CHC for 10 years or more (Havrilesky, 2013). This protection continues for at least 30 years after discontinuation.
- Reduction in functional ovarian cysts and fibroid formation.
- Reduces risk of endometrial cancer; this risk reduction correlates with duration of use. After 10–15 years of use the risk is reduced by 50% and there is persistence of this protective effect for up to 30 years after cessation of use.
- Incidence of bowel cancer is reduced by 19%. However, longer duration of use does not appear to confer greater reduction in risk.
- Continuous CHC use can improve the symptoms of endometriosis and can reduce risk of recurrence of endometriosis after surgical management.
- Helps to protect against pelvic inflammatory disease.
- Can be used for management of acne, hirsutism and menstrual irregularities associated with polycystic ovary syndrome.
- Menopausal symptoms may be reduced. Extended use or a reduced pill-free interval may further improve symptom control.

4.5.2 Disadvantages

- These methods must be used correctly and consistently to be effective.
- Drug interactions reduce efficacy.
- Patches cause local skin reaction in up to 20% of users.
- Vaginal ring causes 'vaginitis' in 5–14% of women.
- CHC does not provide protection against STIs.
- There is a small increased risk of breast cancer in current CHC users. This risk may increase with duration of use. The risk declines gradually after stopping CHC use, returning to the same risk as never user of CHC by 5–10 years of non-use.
- After 5 years of use, these methods may be associated with an increase in the incidence of cervical intraepithelial neoplasia (CIN) and cancer of the cervix. The combined hormonal components appear to be a co-factor leading to persistence or repeated replication of oncogenic human papilloma virus. Those taking CHC should be advised to have regular cervical screening as indicated by the NHS cervical screening programme (NHSCSP). Women who have previously been treated for CIN may choose to take a CHC because the benefits outweigh the potential risks. They should be advised to continue cervical screening as indicated by the NHSCSP.
- There is an increased risk of MI in CHC users. The absolute risk from a Danish cohort study was 1.0 per 10 000 woman-years of use of hormonal contraception. This risk

is increased in women who smoke (up to 20-fold increased risk) and in those with hypertension.

- There is a small increased risk of ischaemic stroke in current CHC users. The absolute risk from a Danish cohort study was 2.1 per 10 000 woman-years of use of hormonal contraception. The risk of ischaemic stroke is increased further in women who experience migraine with aura, from an odds ratio of 2.7 with no CHC use to an odds ratio of 6.1 with CHC use. There is no increased risk of haemorrhagic stroke associated with CHC use.
- Current use of CHC is associated with increased risk of VTE from a baseline of approximately 2 in 10 000 to 5–12 in 10 000. This risk of VTE is highest in the months immediately after initiation or when restarting after a break of at least 1 month. The risk then reduces over the first year of use and thereafter remains stable. Some CHC formulations are associated with a greater risk of VTE than others (see *Table 4.2*); the various progestogens may modify the effect of oestrogen on hepatic clotting factors in different ways.

Table 4.2 Risk of developing a VTE in a year

Women **not using** a combined hormonal pill/patch/ring and who are not pregnant	About 2 out of 10 000 women
Women who are pregnant or in the immediate post-partum period	About 29 out of 10 000 women
Women using a CHC containing **levonorgestrel, norethisterone or norgestimate**	About 5–7 out of 10 000 women
Women using a CHC containing **etonogestrel or norelgestromin**	About 6–12 out of 10 000 women
Women using a CHC containing **drospirenone, gestodene or desogestrel**	About 9–12 out of 10 000 women
Women using a CHC containing **dienogest or nomegestrol acetate**	Not yet known

Data from MHRA (2014); SPC for oestradiol valerate and dienogest (2018) and SPC for oestradiol hemihydrate and nomegestrol acetate (2019).

4.6 Using the CHC

- Prior to starting the CHC, medical eligibility needs to be determined from medical, drug (including over-the-counter preparations), family and lifestyle histories (see *Chapters 2* and *3*). Documentation of blood pressure and BMI is recommended.
- If medically eligible, a discussion of the effectiveness, benefits, risks, side-effects and advice regarding when to stop the CHC or seek medical review is advised. This discussion should be supplemented by the provision of written information or a trusted internet link (such as www.sexwise.fpa.org.uk/contraception) to support CHC use.
- A good first-line CHC is one containing ≤30 micrograms ethinylestradiol in combination with levonorgestrel or norethisterone.

- Women wishing to use the CHC as their method of contraception should be provided with information about standard and tailored regimes, to enable them to make a decision about the most appropriate regimen for them.
- A prescription for up to a 12-month supply of CHC can be provided, whether initiating or continuing this method based on clinical assessment. For some women it may be of benefit to provide CHC for a shorter duration of 3 or 6 months between reviews. The CVR can only be prescribed 1 pack or three months at a time, therefore arrangements will be required for women to obtain repeat prescriptions without the need for 3-monthly medical review.

4.6.1 Standard use

- For most preparations the CHC is taken daily for 21 days followed by a 7 day pill-free or placebo pill interval, during which time a withdrawal bleed will occur. Apps are available to help users remember to take their pills. There are a small number of COCs with 24 active pills and 4 placebo pills.
- The CTP is changed every 7 days for 3 weeks followed by a patch-free week.
- The CVR is inserted into the vagina and remains in place for 3 weeks followed by a ring-free week.
- All of the methods have similar efficacy, but the CTP and CVR are advantageous for women who cannot remember a daily pill or who have gastrointestinal problems affecting pill absorption.
- The CHCs containing oestradiol and nomegestrol acetate or estetrol and drospirenone include four placebo tablets in each 28 day cycle. Oestradiol valerate and dienogest have a quadriphasic regimen including two placebo tablets in each 28 day cycle. The latter preparation has an oestrogenic step-down and progestogenic step-up dosing regimen, reducing the incidence of breakthrough bleeding associated with oestradiol-containing pills. The oestradiol and nomegestrol acetate and oestradiol valerate and dienogest pills are associated with a shorter withdrawal bleed (3–4 days for the former and 4 days for the latter) compared to other CHCs (typically 5 days). There is a higher likelihood of missing a withdrawal bleed (18–32% for oestradiol and nomegestrol compared to 5% with drospirenone-containing CHCs, and 19.4% for oestradiol valerate and dienogest). A pregnancy test is advised if two withdrawal bleeds are missed.

4.6.2 Tailored use (off licence)

- There is no medical reason to have a monthly withdrawal bleed.

Tailored regimens can reduce the frequency of withdrawal bleeds and can reduce withdrawal symptoms such as headache, bloating, tiredness and menstrual pain, which can occur during the HFI. However, unscheduled bleeding is common. There are four options when it comes to tailoring:

- Shortened HFI – 21 days of active pills or 3 patches or 1 ring are used, followed by a 4-day interval.
- Extended use – wherein the CHC method is used for 9 weeks, i.e. 3 packets of pills, 9 patches or 3 rings. Following this a 7 day or 4 day method-free interval is taken, after which the method is recommenced.
- Alternatively, the chosen CHC method can be used flexibly with continuous use for at least 21 days. Then if troublesome breakthrough bleeding occurs for 3–4 days the CHC can be stopped for an interval of 4 or 7 days. It is then recommended that the CHC is used for at least a further 21 days before another method-free interval is taken.
- Continuous use – when the CHC is used continuously with no HFI.

Multiphasic COC should not be used in tailored regimens.

4.6.3 Vomiting and severe diarrhoea

- Efficacy of CHCs can be affected by vomiting and severe diarrhoea.
- If vomiting occurs within 2 hours of taking the CHC, another pill should be taken and no further action is needed.
- If the vomiting continues or severe diarrhoea occurs it is advisable to follow the missed pills advice (see *Section 4.6.6*).

4.6.4 Drug interactions

- Non-enzyme inducing antibiotics such as amoxycillin do not affect the efficacy of CHCs.
- Liver enzyme inducing drugs such as carbamazepine, phenytoin and topiramate increase the metabolism of both oestrogen and progestogen, thereby reducing the contraceptive efficacy of CHC (see *Chapter 2*). It may be more prudent to change the method of contraception provided for women who are using liver enzyme inducing medication long-term.
- Lamotrigine monotherapy with CHC use may result in a reduction in serum levels of lamotrigine. It could result in an increased seizure frequency during CHC use and toxicity risk during the CHC-free interval. Therefore concomitant use is not recommended as the potential risks outweigh the benefits.
- CHC users should wait 5 days after taking UPA-EC before commencing their CHC. During this time, and until the CHC has become effective, condoms or abstinence will be required.

4.6.5 Starting regimens

These are described in *Table 4.3* below.

Table 4.3 Starting regimens for CHCs

Circumstances	Start when?	Requirement for 7 days of additional contraceptive precautions (9 days for estradiol valerate/dienogest COC)?
Natural menstrual cycle	Up to and including day 5	No
	At any other time if it is reasonably certain she is not pregnant and/or a high sensitivity urine pregnancy test (HSUPT) is negative	Yes
Amenorrhoea	At any time if it is reasonably certain she is not pregnant and/or a HSUPT is negative	Yes
Quick starting	At any time if it is reasonably certain she is not pregnant or a HSUPT is negative (see *Chapter 2*)	Yes
Following childbirth • breastfeeding	From 6 weeks following childbirth	Yes
• not breastfeeding	Without additional risk factors* for VTE – from 3 weeks	Yes
	With additional risk factors* for VTE – from 6 weeks	Yes
Following abortion, miscarriage, ectopic pregnancy or gestational trophoblastic disease	Up to and including day 5 following treatment (day 1 for oestradiol valerate/dienogest)	No
	After day 5 if reasonably certain she is not pregnant (day 1 for oestradiol valerate/dienogest)	Yes
Following oral emergency contraception • after LNG-EC	Immediately	Yes
• after UPA- EC	No sooner than 5 days after taking UPA-EC	Yes
Switching from another CHC	Start on day after last active COC, CVR or CTP or during weeks 2–3 or subsequent consecutive weeks of CHC if using extended regimen	No
	Week 1 or days 3–7 of HFI AND no UPSI since start of HFI	Yes
	Week 1 or days 3–7 of HFI AND UPSI since start of HFI	Continue CHC until 7 consecutive days taken, then advice as for week 2 or 3
		If a HFI is taken, the need for additional precautions or emergency contraception should be individually assessed, taking account of correct use before the HFI

Circumstances	Start when?	Requirement for 7 days of additional contraceptive precautions (9 days for estradiol valerate/dienogest COC)?
Switching from a traditional POP	Can be started immediately if the POP has been used consistently and correctly	Yes
Switching from progestogen-only anovulatory methods • desogestrel pill	Start on day after last desogestrel POP	No
• injectable	Start any time up to when the repeat injection is due	CHC will have suppressed ovulation by the time the inhibitory effect of the previous method is lost
• implant	Start any time up to when the implant is due for removal	
Switching from LNG-IUS	Start at any time	Yes if IUS removed on day of method changed, or No if LNG-IUS remains *in situ* for 7 (or 9) days until the CHC becomes effective If there has been any UPSI in the preceding 7 days the LNG-IUS should be left *in situ* for 7 days
Switching from IUD	Up to day 5 of menstrual cycle (day 1 oestradiol COC)	No
	At any other time during the menstrual cycle	Yes If IUD removed on day of method changed, or No if IUD remains *in situ* for 7 (or 9) days until the CHC becomes effective If there has been any UPSI in the preceding 7 days the IUD should be left *in situ* for 7 days

* other risk factors for VTE: immobility, transfusion at delivery, BMI ≥30 kg/m², post-partum haemorrhage, immediately post-caesarean delivery, pre-eclampsia and smoking.

4.6.6 Advice about missed or late CHC

- A missed pill is one which is taken more than 24 hours after the pill was due but less than 48 hours late (48–72 hours since the last pill was taken).
- It is recommended that women are advised to consider alternative methods if they frequently miss pills or repeatedly make errors while using a patch or ring.
- If one pill is missed, it should be taken as soon as it is remembered and the rest of the pack should be continued. No further action is generally required.
- If two or more pills missed (i.e. more than 72 hours since last pill was taken or more than 48 hours late in restarting pill after pill-free interval) see *Table 4.4* for advice.

Table 4.4 Missed pills advice

Pills missed	Guidance
If two or more pills are missed in the first week or the HFI is extended (>7 days)	• Take most recent missed pill • Continue with the rest of the pack and use condoms or abstain for the next 7 days • If sexual intercourse occurred in the preceding 7 days, emergency contraception may be needed (see *Chapter 13*)
Two or more missed pills and more than 7 pills left in the packet	• Take the most recent missed pill • Continue with the rest of the pack and use condoms or abstain for the next 7 days • Finish packet and have the pill-free interval as usual
Two or more missed pills and less than 7 pills left in the packet	• Take the most recent missed pill • Continue with the rest of the pack and use condoms or abstain for the next 7 days • Omit the pill-free interval, finish the active tablets in the current packet and immediately start a new packet; do not take any of the inactive or placebo tablets

If a CHC containing oestradiol and nomegestrol is taken less than 24 hours late there is no reduction in contraceptive efficacy. If the pill is taken more than 24 hours late see *Table 4.5* for missed pills advice.

If one CHC pill containing oestradiol valerate and dienogest, estetrol and drospirenone, or 20 mcg ethinyl estradiol and drospirenone is taken more than 12 hours late, the missed pills advice in *Table 4.6* is recommended.

Table 4.5 Missed pills advice – oestradiol-, nomegestrol- and estetrol/drospirenone-containing CHCs

When pills missed	Guidance
Day 1–7	• Take the pill when it is remembered, even if it means taking 2 tablets at the same time • Use barrier methods for next 7 days; consider EC
Day 8–17	• 1 tablet missed, take it when remembered, no condoms needed unless other pills have been missed earlier in the pack • >1 tablet missed, use condoms for next 7 days
Day 18–24	Option 1: skip placebo pills, no additional need for condom use providing no missed pills in the preceding 7 days; may get some menstrual spotting
	Option 2: stop taking active pills and take a maximum of 3 days of the placebo tablets so that not more than 4 active tablets are missed; then begin new pack

4.6.7 Advice regarding incorrect use of CTP and CVR

- If the HFI is increased to greater than 7 days, a new patch or ring should be applied or inserted as soon as possible. Additional contraception or abstinence is needed for 7 days. There may be a need for EC if sexual intercourse occurred in the HFI (see *Chapter 13*).

- If the CTP or CVR is detached or removed for less than 48 hours:
  - a new patch should be attached or a ring inserted
  - no additional contraception is required providing the method has been used correctly in the previous 7 days (or earlier in week 1 and in the 7 days prior to the HFI if detachment or removal occurs in week 1 after the HFI).
- If the CTP or CVR is detached or removed for more than 48 hours:
  - a new patch or the ring should be attached or inserted as soon as possible and continued until scheduled change or removal day; additional contraception or abstinence is required for the following 7 days
  - if the removal or detachment occurs in week 1 following the HFI there may be a need for EC if sexual intercourse occurred in the HFI (see *Chapter 13*)
  - if unscheduled removal or detachment occurred in the week prior to a planned HFI, this interval should be omitted and additional contraception or abstinence used for 7 days.
- Continued use of CTP for more than 7 days:
  - if a patch is used for more than 7 but less than 9 days (i.e. up to 48 additional hours), no additional contraception or EC is required, providing that the method has been correctly used for the preceding 7 days or earlier in week 1, and for the week prior to the HFI if the detachment occurs in week 1.
  - if a patch is used for more than 9 days (i.e. more than 48 additional hours) women are advised to apply a new patch, omit the HFI (if within 7 days of the HFI) and use additional contraception or abstinence for the following 7 days.
- Continued use of the CVR for more than 3 weeks:
  - if a ring is used for more than 21 days but less than 28, women can either start their HFI and insert a new ring at the end of the HFI, or insert a new ring and miss the HFI; additional contraception or abstinence is not required, nor is EC, providing the ring was consistently *in situ* from day 21 to day 28
  - if a ring is used for more than 4 weeks but less than 5, women are advised to omit the HFI and insert a new ring; additional contraception or abstinence is needed for 7 days but EC not required if the ring was consistently *in situ* from day 21 to 28 of use

Table 4.6 Missed pills advice – oestradiol valerate- and dienogest-containing CHCs

When pills missed	Guidance
Day 1–17	Take the missed pill as soon as possible, even if it means taking 2 pills at the same time Continue taking pills according normal use Use barrier method for 9 days
Day 18–24	Discard remaining pills, start new packet and take normally Use barrier method for 9 days
Day 25–26	Take the missed pill as soon as possible, even if it means taking 2 pills at the same time No barrier method needed
Day 27–28	Discard missed pill and continue taking the packet as normal; no barrier method needed

- ○ if a ring is used for more than 5 weeks, women are advised to omit the HFI and insert a new ring; additional contraception or abstinence is needed for 7 days. If unprotected sexual intercourse has occurred in week 5 or beyond, EC should be considered (see *Chapter 13*).

4.6.8 Indications that a medical review is needed

Symptoms that require an urgent medical review:
- Calf pain, swelling and/or redness
- Chest pain and/or breathlessness and/or coughing up blood
- Loss of motor or sensory function.

Symptoms that a require a medical review:
- Breast lump, unilateral nipple discharge, new nipple inversion, change in breast skin
- New onset migraine
- New onset sensory or motor symptoms in the hour preceding onset of migraine
- Persistent unscheduled vaginal bleeding.

New medical diagnoses that require advice from contraceptive provider to determine the ongoing suitability of CHC:
- High blood pressure
- High body mass index (>35 kg/m^2)
- Migraine, or migraine with aura
- Deep vein thrombosis or pulmonary embolism
- Blood clotting abnormality
- Antiphospholipid antibodies
- Angina, myocardial infarction, stroke or peripheral vascular disease
- Atrial fibrillation
- Cardiomyopathy
- Breast cancer or breast cancer gene mutation
- Liver tumour
- Symptomatic gallstones.

4.6.9 Surgery and immobility

- VTE risk in CHC users is further increased with prolonged immobility and following major surgery.
- Women should discuss discontinuing the CHC with their surgeon.
- It is normally advised that CHC should be stopped 4 weeks prior to major elective surgery, surgery to the lower limbs, and surgery which will result in prolonged immobility but not for minor or short duration surgery.
- Alternative contraceptive options should be discussed and commenced to avoid unplanned pregnancy. All progestogen-only methods are suitable in this situation.
- The CHC can be recommenced at least 2 weeks after full mobilization.

4.7 Routine follow-up

- Reassess medical eligibility and review current medication, method adherence and satisfaction. In addition, blood pressure and BMI are recorded or can be self-reported by women if consultations are online or by phone.
- Women are advised to return at any time if they have concerns or are experiencing troubling side-effects, have changes in their general health, commence new medication, wish to discontinue CHC or to discuss alternative methods.
- CHCs can be used during the peri-menopause in non-smoking women with no other contraindications and may reduce menopausal symptoms, especially if the HFI is reduced.
- CHCs can be continued until the age of 50 after which an alternative method is advised. This should be continued until the age of 55 years by which time 98% of women will be at least 1 year past their last menstrual period (see *Chapter 2*).

4.8 Return to fertility

- There is no delay in return to fertility and increasing duration of use is not associated with reduced fertility.
- The earliest estimated date of ovulation following missed combined pills or cessation of CHC is 10 days. Typically, ovulation occurs within 1 month of stopping CHC use.
- Conception rate is 79.4–95.0% within 12 months of ceasing CHC use.

4.9 Managing side-effects

Unscheduled bleeding is one of the most common side-effects, reported by approximately 20% of CHC users. This generally resolves over the first 3 months of use.

If bleeding persists and other pathology known to cause IMB, such as STI, pregnancy, cervical pathology and missed pills, has been excluded, consider increasing the oestrogen dose to ≥30 micrograms or change the progestogen to a second generation or a trial of the CVR (increased bioavailability of the steroids via this route of administration). Explain that there is an element of trial and error to find the right choice for each woman.

Side-effects such as headaches, genital irritation, tiredness, bloating and menstrual pain may occur in the HFI rather than during active pill use. Extended, continuous use or shortening the pill-free interval may be beneficial.

Hormonally-associated side-effects include:
- **Nausea** – taking the pill at night may improve symptoms; alternatively a CVR or CTP could also be tried.
- **Breast tenderness** – a support bra or evening primrose oil for cyclical pain may be tried prior to a change in CHC.
- **Chloasma** (skin discolouration) – the use of skin block is recommended in conjunction with stopping the CHC and changing to POP, although it may continue with POP.

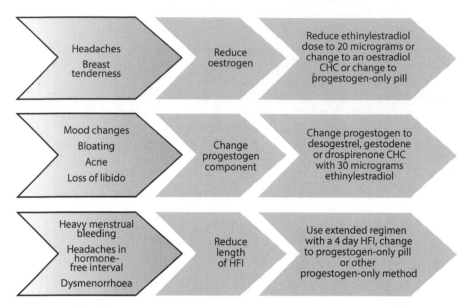

Figure 4.1 Side-effect management options.

- **Acne** – lifestyle, diet and skin care advice are an initial management approach. If acne continues, change progestogen to desogestrel, gestodene or drospirenone CHC with 30 micrograms ethinylestradiol. If it continues after 3 months add in topical or systemic acne treatment. If acne fails to improve after 6 months, change to cyproterone acetate and 35 micrograms ethinylestradiol.
- **Hirsutism** – change to a drospirenone with 30 micrograms ethinylestradiol CHC. If there is little response after 6 months, change to cyproterone acetate and 35 micrograms ethinylestradiol.
- **Mood changes and loss of libido** – in addition to considering a change in progestogen it is important to explore relationship and personal issues.

There is no clear, consistent evidence that CHC use causes depression; if negative mood changes are experienced but the CHC is still the desired method of contraception, different progestogens could be tried. In addition there is no clear evidence of an association between use of CHC containing ≥20 micrograms ethinylestradiol and libido.

CTP-specific side-effects include application site skin reaction in up to 20% of women. These reactions include irritation, redness, itch or rash. If they occur the patch should be removed and a new patch applied to another site. Skin reactions are an infrequent reason for discontinuation (2.6%).

CVR-specific side-effects include vaginitis (5.6%), change in vaginal discharge (4.8%) and awareness of the CVR during sexual intercourse (reported by 18% of women and 32% of partners). Foreign body sensation, coital problems and ring expulsion are less common, collectively affecting 4.4% of users.

4.10 Myths and misconceptions

- **CHCs should be stopped after 5 years of use** – there is no medical reason to support women taking a break. Women who take a break and remain sexually active increase their risk of pregnancy. Taking a break from the CHC for 1 month or more then re-starting increases the risk of IMB and more significantly VTE. Additionally, the CHC has a duration-related protective effect for ovarian and endometrial cancer which supports continuation.
- **CHCs cause weight gain** – there is no evidence that CHCs cause weight gain. Weight fluctuates naturally due to changes in age or life circumstance; women tend to gain weight as they age. In addition, most evidence suggests no association between weight/body mass index (BMI) and effectiveness of CHCs. However, there is limited evidence to suggest a possible reduction in patch effectiveness in women ≥90 kg.
- **CHCs reduce sexual desire and pleasure** – there is no evidence that CHCs affect a woman's sex drive.
- **CHCs cause acne** – although it is a common belief that CHCs cause acne, evidence suggests that CHCs may reduce acne lesions and those containing cyproterone acetate are licensed to treat severe acne.
- **CHCs must be stopped before air travel** – long-haul travel is a moderate risk factor for VTE. It is advisable that women keep well hydrated, avoid alcohol and undertake appropriate exercise to reduce immobility. Experts recommend that women who are spending more than one week at altitudes above 4500m should consider avoiding CHC. Below this altitude, use of CHC is likely to be safe in a healthy, non-smoking woman.

EXAMPLE

A 27 year old attends for review to discuss irregular bleeding with her combined pill. She has taken it for 9 months.

What questions do you ask her? What are her contraceptive options if she wishes to continue to use a CHC?

1. Check compliance, pregnancy risk, malabsorption, drug interactions and undertake an STI risk assessment.
2. Check she has had a cervical screen within the last 3 years.
3. The CVR provides the best cycle control, with irregular bleeding occurring in just 2% of users compared to 39% in pill users. If she wishes to continue with a pill then 30 micrograms ethinylestradiol and 75 micrograms gestodene, or 35 micrograms ethinylestradiol and 250 micrograms norgestimate would be good alternatives.
4. Alternatively she may wish to try a LARC.

References

British National Formulary, March 2023–September 2023.

EMC (2018) *Qlaira Film-Coated Tablets* (oestradiol valerate dienogest): Summary of product characteristics.
[www.medicines.org.uk/emc/product/6536/smpc – accessed May 2023]

EMC (2019) *Zoely 2.5 mg/1.5 mg Film-Coated Tablets* (oestradiol hemihydrate nomegestrol acetate): Summary of product characteristics.
[www.medicines.org.uk/emc/product/3038/smpc – accessed May 2023]

FSRH (2019, amended 2020) *Combined Hormonal Contraception*. Clinical Effectiveness Unit.
[www.fsrh.org/standards-and-guidance/documents/combined-hormonal-contraception – accessed May 2023]

FSRH (2020, amended 2021) *Recommended Actions after Incorrect Use of Combined Hormonal Contraception (e.g. late or missed pills, ring and patch)*. Clinical Effectiveness Unit.
[www.fsrh.org/standards-and-guidance/documents/fsrh-ceu-guidance-recommended-actions-after-incorrect-use-of – accessed May 2023]

Havrilesky, L.J. *et al.* (2013) Oral contraceptive pills as primary prevention for ovarian cancer: a systematic review and meta-analysis. *Obstetrics and Gynaecology*, 122 (1): 139–47.

Lidegaard, Ø., Løkkegaard, E., Jensen, A. *et al.* (2012) Thrombotic stroke and myocardial infarction with hormonal contraception. *New England Journal of Medicine*, **366**: 2257–66.

MHRA (2014) Drug Safety Update: *Combined hormonal contraceptives and venous thromboembolism: review confirms risk is small*.
[www.gov.uk/drug-safety-update/combined-hormonal-contraceptives-and-venous-thromboembolism-review-confirms-risk-is-small – accessed May 2023]

NICE (2019, updated 2021) NG88: *Heavy Menstrual Bleeding*.
[www.nice.org.uk/guidance/ng88 – accessed May 2023]

Tepper, N.K., Whiteman, M.K., Zapata, L.B. *et al.* (2016) Safety of hormonal contraceptives among women with migraine: a systematic review. *Contraception*, **94**: 630–40.

UKMEC (2016) *UK Medical Eligibility Criteria for Contraceptive Use*
[www.fsrh.org/ukmec – accessed May 2023]

Chapter 5
Progestogen-only pill

The progestogen-only pill (POP) is taken by about 6% of women aged 16–49 years in the UK, although it is less popular in other European countries. Almost half of the prescriptions in 2020 for oral contraception were for a POP. A desogestrel POP is now available to buy from pharmacies.

5.1 Potential users

5.1.1 Most appropriate users

Almost all women who require contraception can take a POP.

5.1.2 Not suitable for the following users

The POP may not be effective in women taking liver enzyme inducing drugs and should be avoided in women who:
- have had a hormone-dependent tumour (e.g. breast cancer) in the last 5 years
- have severe decompensating cirrhosis or liver tumours
- are sensitive to any of the components of the POP
- are currently taking a POP and develop ischaemic heart or cerebrovascular disease.

Generic desogestrel POPs contain soybean oil and are contraindicated in those with a peanut allergy. Branded tablets such as Cerazette, Cerelle and Zelleta should be prescribed by name, as they do not contain this oil. All oral COCs and POPs contain lactose as an excipient in a small dose and should not affect most women unless they have severe lactose intolerance.

5.2 Available POPs in the UK

These are listed in *Table 5.1*.

Table 5.1 POPs currently available in the UK

Trade name	Progestogen and dose	Price (NHS indicative price)
Noriday	Norethisterone 350 micrograms	84 tablets Drug tariff £2.10 (£2.10)
Norgeston	Levonorgestrel 30 micrograms	35 tablets Drug tariff £0.92 (£0.92)
Cerazette	Desogestrel 75 micrograms	84 tablets Drug tariff £2.36 (£9.55)
Cerelle		84 tablets Drug tariff £2.36 (£4.30)
Desogestrel generic		84 tablets Drug tariff £2.36 (varies)
Dosomono		84 tablets Drug tariff £2.36 (£6.50)
Desorex		84 tablets Drug tariff £2.36 (£2.45)
Feanolla		84 tablets Drug tariff £2.36 (£3.49)
Zelleta		84 tablets Drug tariff £2.36 (£2.98)

Data from *BNF*, 2023.

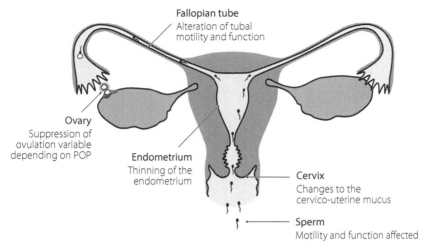

Figure 5.1 Mechanism of action for POPs.

5.3 Mechanism of action

The mechanisms of action are illustrated in *Figure 5.1*.
- Ovulation may be suppressed in up to 60% of cycles by POPs containing levonorgestrel or norethisterone, but in up to 97–99% by those containing desogestrel.
- All POPs alter the cervical mucus to reduce sperm penetration into the upper genital tract.
- POPs induce changes in the endometrium to prevent sperm survival and implantation of the blastocyst.
- Sperm motility and function is affected, preventing fertilization.

5.4 Efficacy of POPs

The POP is very effective when taken consistently and correctly; with 'perfect use' the failure rate is less than 1%. However, the typical failure rate is 7% in the first year of use (see *Table 1.1*). The desogestrel POP is first line for most women as it is thought to be more effective than traditional POPs (as it usually inhibits ovulation and has a 12 rather than 3 hour safety window), but this has not been shown in any published study.

5.5 Pros and cons of POPs

5.5.1 Advantages

- Unrelated to sexual intercourse.
- Simple, convenient to use, and under the woman's control.
- Can be taken when breastfeeding.
- May help to reduce dysmenorrhoea and also the severity of migraines.
- Ideal for women who suffer from oestrogenic side-effects when using CHC, e.g. breast tenderness, headaches including migraines, fluid retention, leg cramps or nausea.

- Suitable for women over 35 years who smoke.
- Can be used in overweight or obese women with no dose adjustment.
- Can be taken by those with medical illnesses where CHCs are contraindicated, e.g. women with hypertension, migraine with focal aura, or with a previous personal history of VTE.
- No evidence of an increased risk of cardiovascular disease, thromboembolism or stroke.
- Minimal alteration in carbohydrate and lipid metabolism, therefore a useful option for diabetics, even those with neuropathic or nephropathic complications.

5.5.2 Disadvantages

- Some women complain of nuisance side-effects such as breast tenderness, mood changes, headaches or acne.
- Overall risk of pregnancy is reduced when taking a POP, but 1 in 10 of these pregnancies may be ectopic in traditional POP users.
- Can alter ovulation, thereby disrupting the menstrual bleeding pattern, with users reporting increased breakthrough bleeding, spotting and amenorrhoea.
- Functional ovarian cysts may develop in a small number of women; however, these tend to be transient and rarely require surgical intervention.

5.6 Using the POP

The POP is taken every day with no break. Following oral ingestion the effect on the cervical mucus reaches its peak within 2–3 hours then slowly wanes over the next 22 or so hours. POPs containing desogestrel differ from more traditional POPs because the main mode of action is to inhibit ovulation and so these POPs have a 12 hour rather than a 3 hour safety window. Women who normally take their traditional POP at 8 am have up to 11 am that day to take their pill. Those taking a desogestrel POP have until 8 pm that night (see advice on missed pills in *Section 5.6.2*).

The efficacy of the POP may be affected by vomiting or severe diarrhoea:
- If vomiting occurs within 2 hours of taking the POP, another pill is taken and no further action is required.
- If vomiting continues and/or an individual is 3 or more hours later than normal taking the pill (12 hours for a desogestrel POP), then the missed pill guidance should be followed.

The efficacy of the POP can be affected by concomitant use of a liver enzyme inducing drug, such as carbamazepine, phenobarbital, phenytoin, topiramate, rifabutin, rifampicin, some antiretrovirals, ulipristal acetate, bosentan, St John's wort and possibly lamotrigine.
- When these drugs are used short term, an additional method such as condoms should be used during the time of drug administration and for 4 weeks after stopping the medication.
- An alternative method such as an injectable or intrauterine contraceptive should be chosen if the liver enzyme inducing drug is to be used long term.

5.6.1 Starting regimens

These are described in *Table 5.2* below.

Table 5.2 Starting regimens for POPs

Circumstances	Start when?	Requirement for 2 days (48 hours) of additional contraceptive precautions?
Natural menstrual cycle	Up to and including day 5	No
	At any other time if it is reasonably certain she is not pregnant and/or a high sensitivity urine pregnancy test (HSUPT) is negative	Yes
Amenorrhoea	At any time if it is reasonably certain she is not pregnant and/or HSUPT is negative	Yes
Quick starting	At any time if it is reasonably certain she is not pregnant or a HSUPT is negative (see *Chapter 2*)	Yes
Following childbirth (breastfeeding and non-breastfeeding)	Up to day 21 post-partum	No
	After day 21 post-partum	Yes (unless using LAM)
Following abortion, miscarriage, ectopic pregnancy or gestational trophoblastic disease	Day 1–5	No
	After day 5 if it is reasonably certain she is not pregnant	Yes
Following oral emergency contraception		
• after LNG-EC	Immediately	Yes
• after UPA- EC	No sooner than 5 days after taking UPA-EC	Yes
Switching from another POP	At any time	No
Switching from a CHC	Day 1–2 of HFI	No
	Day 3–7 of HFI or week 1 following	Yes If UPSI has occurred after day 3 of HFI advise continuing CHC for 7 days
	Week 2–3 of CHC	No, providing the method has been used consistently and correctly prior to switching
Switching from progestogen-only anovulatory methods		
• injectable	Start any time up to when repeat injection is due	No
• implant	Start any time up to when implant is due for removal	No

(continued)

Circumstances	Start when?	Requirement for 2 days (48 hours) of additional contraceptive precautions?
Switching from LNG-IUS	Start at any time	Yes if IUS removed on day of method changed, or
		No if LNG-IUS remains *in situ* for 2 days until the POP becomes effective
		If there has been any UPSI in the preceding 7 days the LNG-IUS should be left *in situ* for 7 days
Switching from IUD	Day 1–5 of cycle	No
	After day 5 of cycle	Yes if IUD removed on day of method changed, or
		No if IUD remains *in situ* for 2 days until the POP becomes effective
		If there has been any UPSI in the preceding 7 days the IUD should be left *in situ* for 7 days

5.6.2 Advice about missed pills

- POPs are effective if taken consistently and correctly.
- If less than 3 hours has elapsed from the usual administration/ingestion time for a norethisterone or levonorgestrel-containing POP and less than 12 hours for a desogestrel-containing pill, the missed pill should be taken and the pack continued as normal. No additional cover (e.g. condoms) is required.
- If more than 3 hours has elapsed from the normal administration time (12 hours for desogestrel POP) then the last missed pill is taken, the pack continued as normal, but condoms should also be used as additional contraception for the next 48 hours.
- If more than 3 hours has elapsed from the normal administration time (12 hours for desogestrel POP) and unprotected sex has occurred, emergency contraception should be considered (see *Chapter 13*).

5.7 Routine follow-up

Women can be prescribed or provided with up to a 12-month supply of POP if there are no concerns. Earlier review may be required if nuisance side-effects or compliance concerns are present. POPs can be continued until the age of 55 when 98% of women are at least 1 year after their last natural period. For additional information see *Chapter 3*.

5.8 Return to fertility

There is no delay in return to fertility. Most women ovulate within 2–3 weeks of discontinuing POPs.

5.9 Managing side-effects

Non-specific symptoms such as headache, fatigue and mood change are common in the general population. Treatment-associated serious adverse reactions are very rare with POPs but an irregular bleeding pattern is common and some patients report possible progestogen-associated side-effects.

- In women taking traditional POPs bleeding is unpredictable: 20% will have no periods, 40% irregular bleeding and 40% will have regular cycles. Those taking desogestrel rather than traditional POPs are more likely to have no or infrequent periods after 1 year of use.
- Encourage women to continue with the method for at least 3 months. In those with persistent troublesome bleeding, check compliance and drug interactions, exclude any STIs and pregnancy, examine the cervix and perform cervical cytology if due. Consider a change in POP or contraceptive method.
- Progestogen-associated side-effects may include acne, bloating, mood change and loss of libido. Again, encourage women to continue with the method for at least 3 months. If symptoms persist consider changing the POP to a different progestogen or consider a different method.
- There is no evidence that POPs increase or decrease weight.

5.10 Myths and misconceptions

- **POPs are not very effective in women weighing over 70 kg and these women need to take 2 POPs daily** – there is no evidence that POPs are less effective in overweight or obese women and so standard dosing regimens should be followed.
- **Women taking POPs and having amenorrhoea will have problems getting pregnant** – some women will not bleed while taking a POP. The endometrium is thin and atrophic. This is seen as an additional benefit, with many reporting reduced period pain too. On discontinuation of the POP most women ovulate within the first 3 weeks and menstruate within the next 6 weeks. The POP has no long-term effect on fertility.
- **Women with migraine with aura cannot take POPs** – this is not true. In fact many women with migraine with aura choose to take a POP for contraception because it may help reduce the intensity and frequency of the headaches and aura.

EXAMPLE

An 18 year old woman presents with painful, heavy periods; she also needs contraception. She would like to take the COC. History-taking establishes that her father experienced an unprovoked VTE at the age of 38 years, but there is no other family history of VTE. The family were genetically screened because her father was found to have factor V Leiden; only her sister was found to carry the gene for factor V Leiden.

What do you advise?

1. Using UKMEC this family history suggests that the risks of taking a COC outweigh any potential benefits (UKMEC 3), even though her thrombophilia screen was normal. This is because we can only look for known mutations and she may carry an increased VTE risk from an unknown alteration in genetic sequencing. This should be explained to the patient.
2. Alternatives with a lower risk for this woman would be a desogestrel POP, etonogestrel implant, DMPA or a LNG-IUS.

References

British National Formulary, March 2023–September 2023.

FSRH (2017, amended 2019) *Contraception for Women Aged Over 40*. Clinical Effectiveness Unit.
[www.fsrh.org/standards-and-guidance/documents/fsrh-guidance-contraception-for-women-aged-over-40-years-2017 – accessed May 2023]

FSRH (2022) *Progestogen-only Pills*. Clinical Effectiveness Unit.
[www.fsrh.org/documents/cec-guideline-pop – accessed May 2023]

Office for National Statistics (2009) Opinions Survey Report No. 41 *Contraception and Sexual Health*, 2008/09.

UKMEC (2016) *UK Medical Eligibility Criteria for Contraceptive Use*
[www.fsrh.org/standards-and-guidance/documents/ukmec-2016-summary-sheets/ – accessed May 2023]

Chapter 6

Injectable contraception

Progestogen-only injectables have been available for over 40 years and have a good safety record. About 3% of UK women aged between 16 and 49 years of age use a progestogen-only injectable as their method of contraception, with most users receiving depot medroxyprogesterone acetate (DMPA). Monthly combined injectables containing oestrogen and progestogens are available in some countries outside of Europe. This chapter will discuss progestogen-only injectables, focusing on those containing medroxyprogesterone acetate.

6.1 Potential users

6.1.1 Most appropriate users

Injectable contraceptives can be used by women of reproductive age up to the age of 50 years. For women with no contraindications and who would prefer to continue, injectables can be used up to the age of the menopause when the benefits outweigh the potential risks of use.

6.1.2 Not suitable for the following users

Injectable contraceptives are not suitable for women with:
- cardiovascular or cerebrovascular disease
- significant multiple risk factors for arterial cardiovascular disease
- current or recent breast cancer
- severe decompensating cirrhosis or liver tumours
- unexplained vaginal bleeding
- a high risk of developing osteoporosis.

6.2 Available injectables in the UK

Details of these are listed in *Table 6.1*.

6.3 Mechanism of action

- The main mode of action of DMPA and NET-EN is to inhibit ovulation by suppressing luteinizing hormone (LH) and, to a certain extent, follicle-stimulating hormone (FSH).
- Injectables also alter the cervical mucus, preventing sperm penetration into the upper genital tract.
- Injectables prevent implantation by inducing endometrial atrophy.
- Like other progestogens, injectables modify sperm function and motility.

6.4 Efficacy of injectables

Progestogen-only injectables are highly effective when women receive them on a regular basis, with fewer than 4 women becoming pregnant out of every 1000 over a

Table 6.1 Injectables available in the UK

Injectable	Contents	Injection interval and site	Cost per injection
Depo-Provera	Depot medroxyprogesterone acetate (DMPA) 150 mg (as aqueous suspension); should be shaken vigorously prior to use	Given as a deep intramuscular injection every 12 weeks, normally in the upper outer quadrant of the gluteal region. Other administration sites include lateral thigh and deltoid muscle of upper arm.	£6.01
Sayana Press	DMPA 104 mg (as aqueous suspension); should be shaken vigorously prior to use	Given subcutaneously every 13 weeks in anterior thigh or lower abdomen. It is licensed for pharmacy/self-administration.	£6.90
Noristerat	Norethisterone enanthate (NET-EN) 200 mg (oily injection); should be warmed prior to use	• Given as a deep intramuscular injection every 8 weeks • For short-term, interim contraception but is used infrequently in the UK	£4.05

Data from *BNF*, 2023.

2 year period. With imperfect use the typical failure rate in the general population can be as high as 4 in 100 women over 1 year.

6.5 Pros and cons of injectables

6.5.1 Advantages

- A very effective and discreet method of contraception.
- Sayana Press can be self-administered after appropriate training and supervision.
- If pregnancy was to occur during DMPA use there is no evidence of harm to the pregnancy or fetus.
- Non-intercourse related contraceptive method.
- Very safe with no reported attributable deaths.
- Safe for breastfeeding mothers.
- Can be used in women with sickle cell disease with possible reduction in sickle crisis pain.
- Helpful for women with ovulation pain.
- Most women will have infrequent or no periods after 1 year of use and so it is often used for treatment of heavy menstrual bleeding and pain associated with endometriosis.
- Offers most of the non-contraceptive benefits of CHCs, including protection against pelvic inflammatory disease, extra-uterine pregnancies, functional ovarian cysts and fibroid formation.
- May reduce risk of ovarian and endometrial cancer.
- Minimal metabolic effects occur.

6.5.2 Disadvantages

- A significant number of women fail to return for their second injection, with up to 50% discontinuing injectable use in the first year. Pre-injection counselling is important to give a realistic picture of potential side-effects, especially menstrual bleeding pattern changes in the first 6–12 months.
- The first few injections of DMPA often cause irregular, prolonged vaginal bleeding with increasing episodes of infrequent or no bleeding over time. About one-third of women experience prolonged bleeding (more than 10 days) after receiving their first injection, but 55% are amenorrhoeic at 1 year and 68% at 2 years.
- A possible increase in HIV acquisition/transmission in DMPA users cannot be ruled out and so correct and consistent use of condoms is advised for women at high risk of HIV.
- Weight gain is reported in about one-third of women. Obese adolescents (BMI >30 kg/m^2) are more likely to gain weight. In practice this weight gain is seen within the first 6 months of method use and continues over time. On average women may gain up to 3 kg over the first 2 years.
- Some women may complain of mood changes, headaches, loss of libido, bloating and breast tenderness although no causal association has been found.
- It can cause a short delay in the return to a woman's normal fertility.
- There is a possible small increase in the risk of breast cancer diagnosed within the first few years of DMPA use, but this appears to return to background levels following 5 years or more of use. This finding is likely to be due to a screening bias.
- There is a possible increase in the risk of cervical cancer in long-term DMPA users, but this could be due to confounding lifestyle issues.
- Injectables are given intramuscularly or subcutaneously and cannot be removed if side-effects occur.
- Injection site reactions are more common with subcutaneous DMPA compared to intramuscular DMPA. Up to 9% of women using subcutaneous DMPA reported indurations, scarring and dimpling (fat atrophy) at the injection site. If these occur move to IM injection or another contraceptive method. A small number of women complain of local redness, pain and bruising with either product. Haematoma and abscess formation are rare events.
- DMPA use results in a small reduction of bone mineral density (BMD), similar to fully breastfeeding for 6 months, which recovers gradually on discontinuation. There is no good data suggesting that DMPA causes osteoporosis or bone fracture. Recent data has suggested that DMPA users are at increased risk of fracture **before** they receive their first injection, implying inherent confounders in those using this method. On discontinuation in adults, BMD recovers to a similar level to never users within 3–5 years. In women under 18 years, BMD recovers more rapidly, with it returning to a similar level to never users approximately 18 months after stopping. There is no evidence that routinely giving 'add-back' oestrogen to DMPA users or undertaking additional investigations are warranted.

Advice from the MHRA (Department of Health Medicines and Healthcare Products Regulatory Agency) in 2004 stated:

- In adolescents, DMPA may be used as first-line contraception after other methods have been discussed with the patient and considered to be unsuitable or unacceptable.
- In women of all ages, careful re-evaluation of the risks and benefits of treatment should be carried out every 2 years in those who wish to continue its use.
- In women with significant lifestyle and/or medical risk factors for osteoporosis, other methods of contraception should be considered.

6.6 Using injectables

DMPA is given every 13 weeks and a review undertaken at least every 2 years to assess if there have been any changes in the medical history. DMPA can be used until the age of 50 years when a woman may choose an alternative method if there are concerns about her bone health (see *Section 3.2*). On discontinuation it may take up to 12 months before regular menstrual cycles restart.

There is no evidence that liver enzyme inducing drugs affect the efficacy of DMPA and the injection interval does not need to be shortened. DMPA may interact with ulipristal acetate when prescribed for emergency contraception or the treatment of fibroids, and vice versa. Therefore DMPA should be avoided in those taking ulipristal acetate to treat uterine fibroids. If ulipristal acetate has been taken for emergency contraception, DMPA should not be administered for 5 days. Additional contraceptive precautions should be used for these 5 days and for the next 7 days after the injection has been given (see *Chapter 13*).

Increasing weight or BMI has not been shown to affect DMPA efficacy. In obese women, deltoid or subcutaneous DMPA administration may be preferred.

6.6.1 Starting regimen

The starting regimen is set out in *Table 6.2*.

6.6.2 Advice about late injections

Recent guidance states that both Depo-Provera and Sayana Press can be administered every 13 weeks. No action is required for either preparation until 14 weeks or more has lapsed since the last injection.
- If a woman presents within 14 weeks of receiving her last injection then the next injection is administered and no further action needs to be taken.
- If more than 14 weeks has elapsed since the last injection, but no unprotected sex has occurred from 14 weeks onwards, the next injection is given and additional contraception or abstinence advised for the next 7 days.
- If more than 14 weeks has elapsed since the last injection, and unprotected sex **has only** occurred in the last 5 days, exclude the risk of pregnancy, consider emergency contraception, give the next injection and advise additional

contraception or abstinence for the next 7 days. A pregnancy test should be repeated in 3 weeks.

- If more than 14 weeks has elapsed since the last injection, and unprotected sex has occurred from 14 weeks onwards for more than 5 days, then pregnancy should be excluded, the next injection may be given with additional contraception or abstinence for the next 7 days. A further pregnancy test is advised in 3 weeks. Alternatively a bridging method may be selected until pregnancy can be excluded.

Table 6.2 Starting regimen for injectables

Circumstances	Start when?	Requirement for 7 days of additional contraceptive precautions?
Natural menstrual cycle	Up to and including day 5	No
	At any other time if it is reasonably certain she is not pregnant and/or a high sensitivity urine pregnancy test (HSUPT) is negative	Yes
Amenorrhoea	At any time if it is reasonably certain she is not pregnant and/or HSUPT is negative	Yes
Quick starting	Ideally a bridging method is used in the short term until pregnancy is excluded; however, if this is not acceptable and it is reasonably certain she is not pregnant and/or HSUPT is negative (see *Chapter 2*) the injection may be provided	Yes
Following childbirth	Before and including day 21	No
	After day 21 in women who are menstruating	Yes, as for women having menstrual cycles
	After day 21 in those not menstruating	Yes, as for those women who are amenorrhoeic
Following abortion, miscarriage, ectopic pregnancy or gestational trophoblastic disease	Within 5 days	No
	After 5 days if it is reasonably certain she is not pregnant	Yes
Following oral emergency contraception		
• after LNG-EC	Immediately	Yes
• after UPA- EC	No sooner than 5 days after taking UPA-EC	Yes

Circumstances	Start when?	Requirement for 7 days of additional contraceptive precautions?
Switching from a CHC	Day 1–2 of HFI	No
	Day 3–7 of HFI or week 1 following	Yes
		If UPSI has occurred after day 3 of HFI advise continuing CHC for 7 days
	Week 2–3 of CHC	No, providing the method has been used consistently and correctly prior to switching
Switching from a traditional POP	Start at any time	Yes for 7 days until ovulation suppression can be assured or continue taking POP for a further 7 days
Switching from progestogen-only anovulatory methods		
• desogestrel pill	Start at any time	No
• implant	Start any time up to when implant is due for removal	No
Switching from LNG-IUS	At any time	Yes for 7 days until ovulation suppression can be assured, or No if continue using an IUS for a further 7 days
Switching from IUD	Give the injection up to and including day 5 of cycle; IUD can be removed at the same time	No
	Any other time	Yes if IUD removed on day of method changed, or
		No if IUD remains *in situ* for 7 days until the injection becomes effective
		If there has been any UPSI in the preceding 7 days the IUD should be left *in situ* for 7 days

6.7 Routine follow-up

Women using intramuscular DMPA are advised to return when their next injection is due, unless troublesome side-effects occur, when an earlier appointment is indicated. Those using subcutaneous DMPA are given a year's supply to self-administer with review on an annual basis unless earlier review is required. At that visit enquiries should be made concerning sexual and medical health, changes in bleeding pattern and presence of nuisance side-effects. The MHRA guidance should be followed.

DMPA users are responsible for making repeat appointments but some practices send reminder text messages and others suggest mobile phone apps.

6.8 Return to fertility

There may be a delay to the return of fertility, with mean time to ovulation being 5.3 months after the preceding injection. Fertility rates by 2 years are similar to those discontinuing non-hormonal contraceptive methods.

6.9 Managing side-effects

6.9.1 Prolonged and frequent bleeding

- Women should be counselled about changes in menstrual pattern before DMPA is administered. Prolonged bleeding/spotting is commonly reported during the first injection cycle.
- If prolonged and/or frequent bleeding is reported to be a problem:
  - exclude gynaecological pathology by taking a clinical and lifestyle history enquiring about abdominal/pelvic pain, dyspareunia, vaginal discharge, dysuria, post-coital bleeding, new sexual partners
  - a pelvic examination is required if irregular bleeding has occurred for more than 3 months, other symptoms are present, a previous medical treatment has failed or the woman is anxious
  - exclude pregnancy in sexually active women
  - perform STI screening in those at risk
  - for those eligible to participate in the NHS Cervical Screening programme review cervical screening history and perform a cervical screen only if it is due.
- Treatment may stop a bleeding episode but confers no long-term benefit, including:
  - prescribing a COC (30 micrograms ethinylestradiol with levonorgestrel) for up to 3 months cyclically or continuously (unlicensed), if there are no contraindications. Depending on clinical judgement, it may be used longer term; however, there is no long-term safety data available
  - prescribing tranexamic acid 250 mg four times a day for 5 days or mefenamic acid 500 mg up to three times a day for 5 days to reduce bleeding in the short term
  - reducing the injection interval by 2 weeks if bleeding occurs towards the end of the injection cycle.

6.9.2 Weight gain

- Advise women that two out of three women do not gain weight with DMPA.
- Weight gain with DMPA is more likely to occur in women with a previous history of labile weight changes.
- Keep to a healthy Mediterranean diet containing only complex carbohydrates.
- Women who gain more than 5% of their baseline body weight in the first 6 months are likely to continue to gain weight.

6.10 Myths and misconceptions

- **DMPA reduces your fertility** – DMPA may delay the return of a woman's fertility but does not affect pregnancy rates 2 years after discontinuation.
- **DMPA increases the risk of a premature menopause** – DMPA administration may stop periods but these return within the first year of discontinuation. It does not bring the age of the menopause forward for women.
- **DMPA makes you fat** – there is evidence that some DMPA users gain weight but most either stay the same or lose weight. Those who gain weight often say that they feel hungrier and are therefore eating more. If a woman has a tendency to gain weight then she should be advised to watch her diet when using DMPA. If she gains a significant amount of weight in the first 6 months then she may wish to choose a different method of contraception.
- **DMPA is unsafe as it causes osteoporosis** – there is no evidence that DMPA alone causes osteoporosis or osteoporotic fractures. For the majority of women the change in BMD is of little clinical significance. It is important to take a careful history to exclude any potential risks to bone health before it is prescribed and at 2 yearly intervals.

EXAMPLE

A 24 year old woman has been using DMPA for 3 years. She wants a baby and stopped having DMPA injections 18 months ago but has still not had a period.

What should you do?

1. As it has been 12 months since her last injection, check other causes for secondary amenorrhoea including undertaking blood tests to check FSH, LH, oestradiol, thyroid function tests, prolactin.
2. Check her BMI.
3. Perform a pregnancy test.
4. If all investigations are normal refer her to a gynaecologist who specializes in fertility issues because she may need ovulation induction.

References

British National Formulary, March 2023–September 2023.

eMC: SPC Depo-Provera 150 mg/ml injection
   [www.medicines.org.uk/emc/product/6721/smpc – accessed May 2023]

eMC: SPC Sayana Press 104 mg/0.65 ml suspension for injection
   [www.medicines.org.uk/emc/product/3148/smpc – accessed May 2023]

FSRH (2014, amended 2020) *Progestogen-only Injectable Contraception*. Clinical Effectiveness Unit.
[www.fsrh.org/standards-and-guidance/documents/cec-ceu-guidance-injectables-dec-2014 – accessed May 2023]

FSRH (2015) *Problematic Bleeding with Hormonal Contraception*. Clinical Effectiveness Unit.
[www.fsrh.org/documents/ceuguidanceproblematicbleedinghormonalcontraception – accessed May 2023]

Lanza L.L. *et al.* (2013) Use of depot medroxyprogesterone acetate contraception and incidence of bone fracture. *Obstet Gynecol.* **121:** 593–600.

Office for National Statistics (2009) Opinions Survey Report No. 41 *Contraception and Sexual Health*, 2008/09.

UKMEC (2016) *UK Medical Eligibility Criteria for Contraceptive Use*
[www.fsrh.org/ukmec – accessed May 2023]

Chapter 7
Contraceptive implant

A contraceptive implant offers an alternative way of delivering hormones providing long-acting, low-dose, reversible contraception. It is one of the most effective methods of contraception, it is licensed to provide contraception for 3 years and approximately 2% of women in the UK use this method.

In 1999 a single progestogen-only implant, Implanon, was launched containing 68 mg etonogestrel, the active metabolite of desogestrel. Nexplanon, a bioequivalent implant with additional barium sulphate to make it radiopaque, is now available. Its applicator facilitates single-handed, subdermal insertion.

Norplant, the levonorgestrel implant, consists of six rods inserted subdermally on the inner aspect of the upper arm. It was available in the UK from 1993 until 1999, but UK healthcare professionals may still see women from non-European countries using this multi-rod contraceptive system, or the two-rod levonorgestrel system, Jadelle.

7.1 Potential users

7.1.1 Most appropriate users

There are few contraindications to its use and no age limit so it is suitable for the majority of women.

7.1.2 Not suitable for the following users

The implant may not be effective in women taking liver enzyme inducing drugs and should be avoided in women who:
- have had a hormone-dependent tumour (e.g. breast cancer) in the last 5 years
- have severe decompensating liver disease or liver tumours
- are sensitive to any of the components of the etonogestrel implant
- are currently using an etonogestrel implant and develop ischaemic heart or cerebrovascular disease
- have unexplained vaginal bleeding.

7.2 Available implants in the UK

Nexplanon, which contains 68 mg etonogestrel, is licensed to provide effective contraception for 3 years. It is inserted subdermally on the inner side of the upper arm. It costs £83.43 and is the only implant available in the UK.

7.3 Mechanism of action

- The etonogestrel implant inhibits ovulation by suppressing luteinizing hormone. However, up to 5% of users may ovulate during the third year of use.
- Implants also alter the cervical mucus, inhibiting sperm penetration and thereby preventing fertilization.
- Implants prevent implantation by inducing endometrial atrophy.
- Implants may modify sperm function and motility.

7.4 Efficacy of implants

This is a highly effective method of contraception with less than 1 woman in every 1000 users becoming pregnant over a 3 year period.

Liver enzyme inducing drugs will reduce the efficacy of progestogen implants therefore additional contraception is required when there is concomitant use with certain anti-epileptic medication, ART and enzyme-inducing antibiotics such as rifampicin (see *Chapter 3* for drug interactions).

There have been concerns that progestogen implants are less effective in obese women because etonogestrel levels fall with increasing weight, although they stay within the therapeutic range. While the manufacturer suggests replacing the implant earlier in the third year for such women, there is little evidence to support this. A recent FSRH guideline states that contraceptive implants remain highly effective in women with raised BMI. However, data is lacking on women with BMI ≥40 kg/m². It is a contraceptive method that can safely be used by women who are overweight or obese, and need only be changed every 3 years.

7.5 Pros and cons of contraceptive implants

7.5.1 Advantages

- Long-lasting, effective, immediately reversible contraceptive method.
- It can be used by women who have previously experienced an ectopic pregnancy because it is highly effective and its main mechanism of action is to suppress ovulation. The risk of ectopic pregnancy is very small.
- No effect on future fertility.
- In the rare event of an unplanned pregnancy, there is no evidence of adverse effects on the pregnancy or fetus.
- Non-intercourse related method.
- Free from oestrogen side-effects.
- High user acceptability following pre-insertion counselling, with first year continuation rates of over 70%.
- Requires little medical attention other than at insertion and removal.
- May reduce ovulation pain.
- Reduced incidence of dysmenorrhoea in women with or without endometriosis.
- Reduced total menstrual blood loss in implant users.
- No evidence to suggest adverse effect on bone mineral density.
- Can be used by those where synthetic oestrogen is contraindicated, including women complaining of migraine with aura.
- Does not adversely affect cardiovascular risk factors with no increased risk of VTE, MI or stroke in implant users.
- Has minimal effects on glucose metabolism and liver function.

7.5.2 Disadvantages

- Unpredictable and irregular bleeding patterns are common in implant users, with the bleeding pattern experienced during the first 3 months being broadly predictive of future bleeding patterns.
- In the first two years of implant use, approximately 22% have amenorrhoea, 33% infrequent bleeding, 7% frequent bleeding and 18% prolonged bleeding per 90-day reference period.
- Enlarged ovarian follicles >2.5 cm may be found in 5–25% of implant users. These are rarely symptomatic and tend to disappear over time. Women with persistent follicles are more likely to complain of prolonged bleeding.
- Incidence of progestogen side-effects are similar to other progestogen-only methods and include headache, weight gain, acne, loss of libido, mood changes. No causal association has been found.
- Acne may improve, stay the same or worsen with the use of the implant.
- Fat atrophy may occur over the site of the implant.
- Insertion of implants requires a minor operative procedure under local anaesthetic by trained healthcare professionals.
- Non-palpable implants have been reported in about 1 in 1000 insertions and are related to poor insertion technique. Very occasionally, deep insertion of an implant has resulted in damage to the neurovascular bundle. Referral to an 'expert' centre is advised for implant location using ultrasound scanning or intravascular translocation before removal.
- In cases where the implant cannot be located by ultrasound scanning or X-ray, etonogestrel assays may be required.
- Some women report mild discomfort and bruising following insertion or removal of the implants.
- Infection at the insertion or removal site, irritation over the implant, breakage of the implant, local fibrosis around the implant, migration of the implant and scarring do occur, but only rarely.
- For some women contraceptive implants may not be a suitable method because discontinuation is not under their control.
- There have been no studies looking at progestogen-only implant use and risk of breast cancer and so there is insufficient evidence to indicate any increased risk.
- There have been no studies investigating progestogen-only implant use and gynaecological cancers and so there is insufficient evidence to indicate any increased risk.

7.6 Practical aspects

7.6.1 Implant starting regimen

Table 7.1 provides details as to when implants can be inserted under a range of circumstances.

Table 7.1 Implant starting regimens

Circumstances	Start when?	Requirement for 7 days of additional contraceptive precautions?
Natural menstrual cycle	Up to and including day 5	No
	At any other time if it is reasonably certain she is not pregnant and/or a high sensitivity urine pregnancy test (HSUPT) is negative	Yes
Amenorrhoea	At any time if it is reasonably certain she is not pregnant and/or HSUPT is negative	Yes
Quick starting	At any time if it is reasonably certain she is not pregnant or a HSUPT is negative (see *Chapter 2*)	Yes
Following childbirth	Before and including day 21	No
	After day 21 in women who are menstruating	Yes, as for women having menstrual cycles
	After day 21 in those not menstruating	Yes, as for those women who are amenorrhoeic
Following abortion, miscarriage, ectopic pregnancy or gestational trophoblastic disease	Within 5 days	No
	After 5 days if it is reasonably certain she is not pregnant	Yes
Following oral emergency contraception		
• after LNG-EC	Immediately	Yes
• after UPA- EC	No sooner than 5 days after taking UPA-EC	Yes
Switching from a COC	Day 1–2 of HFI	No
	Day 3–7 of HFI or week 1 following	Yes
		If UPSI has occurred during the HFI advise continuing CHC for 7 days
	Week 2–3 of CHC	No, providing the method has been used consistently and correctly prior to switching
Switching from a traditional POP	Start at any time	Yes for 7 days until ovulation suppression can be assured, or continue taking POP for a further 7 days

(continued)

Circumstances	Start when?	Requirement for 7 days of additional contraceptive precautions?
Switching from progestogen-only anovulatory methods		
• desogestrel pill	Start at any time	No
• injectable	Start any time up to when repeat injection is due (<14 weeks)	No
Switching from LNG-IUS	At any time	Yes for 7 days until ovulation suppression can be assured, or
		No if continue using an IUS for a further 7 days
Switching from IUD	Day 1–5 of cycle	No
	After day 5 of cycle	Yes if IUD removed on day of method changed, or
		No if IUD remains *in situ* for 7 days until the IMP becomes effective
		If there has been any UPSI in the preceding 7 days the IUD should be left *in situ* for 7 days

7.6.2 Insertion of the implant

Those offering implant insertion and removal should be appropriately trained clinicians holding an up-to-date FSRH Letter of Competence in Subdermal Contraceptive Implant Techniques or have equivalent competencies. They should maintain their competence and regularly update their theoretical and practical knowledge.

The location of the insertion is shown in *Figure 7.1* and the basic technique in *Figure 7.2*.
- Etonogestrel implants are either fitted using an aseptic or 'no touch' technique, with the woman either lying down or sitting with her arm resting on a support.
- The non-dominant arm is abducted to 90°, elbow flexed and her hand placed behind her head.
- Local anaesthetic with or without adrenaline is injected subdermally. Addition of a vasoconstrictor reduces blood loss and may be useful in women taking anticoagulants or where removal of a deep implant is planned. Check that the implant is in the insertion needle.
- Insert the implant just under the skin one-third of the way up the inner aspect of the upper arm, over the triceps, 8–10 cm from the medial epicondyle and 3–5 cm posterior to the sulcus of the biceps and triceps (*Figure 7.2*).
- Once the implant has been fitted its position should be confirmed by both the clinician and patient.
  ○ If the implant cannot be felt easily, the woman should be advised to use additional contraception and return in a week when any swelling or bruising

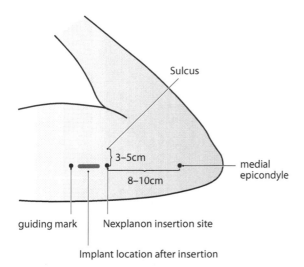

Figure 7.1 Nexplanon insertion site.

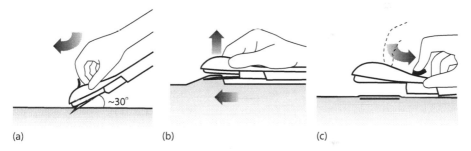

Figure 7.2 Nexplanon insertion. (a) Piercing of the skin; (b) subdermal insertion of the applicator needle, to facilitate placement lift or tent the skin during insertion; (c) retraction of the slider to withdraw the needle, placing the implant subdermally.

following insertion will have resolved. If it is still not palpable then the guidance for managing deep implants (see *Section 7.6.4*) should be followed.

- The applicator is designed to reduce the chance of non-insertion. Following insertion the needle should be fully retracted inside the applicator's handle.
- The arm is then dressed and advice regarding wound care given.

7.6.3 Removal of implant

A woman can decide to have the implant removed at any point following its insertion – she should not be coerced to keep it. Discuss the reasons for its removal and options for treating any side-effects such as erratic bleeding pattern, headaches, etc. Future contraceptive/preconception plans should be covered during the consultation. To avoid an unplanned pregnancy another contraceptive method should be started immediately following removal of the implant (see 'switching advice for individual methods' in *Chapters 4–9*).

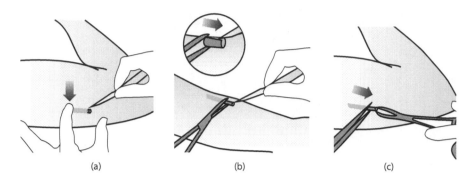

(a)   (b)   (c)

Figure 7.3 Implant removal. (a) Make a small longitudinal incision over the distal end of the implant – the tip of the implant should pop out of the incision; (b) clean away the connective tissue; (c) remove the implant.

The removal procedure is outlined below and illustrated in *Figure 7.3*.
- The skin over the distal end of the implant is marked with water-soluble marker pen and local anaesthetic injected just under its tip.
- A small longitudinal incision is made in the skin and the implant is pushed through the incision using the 'pop out' method.
- Connective tissue is cleaned away from the tip of the implant and the implant is then removed.
- The small wound can be closed with paper strips and then dressed.
- If a further implant is requested, this can be inserted through the same incision, ensuring that its position is subdermal.
- Insertion and removal counselling/procedures should be clearly documented in the clinical record.

7.6.4 Management of deep or bent implants

- Impalpable implants normally result from poor insertion technique and frequently occur at the time of removing and reinserting new implants. Rarely, nerve or vascular damage can occur with deep implant insertions or problematic removals, with intravascular migration to the pulmonary tree occasionally reported. Beware of women with thin arms because the needle tip can be accidentally placed under the muscle fascia, resulting in an intramuscular insertion.
- Implant migration up or down the arm is more commonly seen where the implant is deeply placed in muscle and in women who try to move the implant under their skin.
- If an implant cannot easily be felt then women should be advised to abstain from sex or use an additional method of contraception. In these situations:
  - Do not attempt removal.
  - If the implant is Nexplanon, arrange an X-ray of the arm. If the implant can be seen then it will still be effective as a contraceptive and it does not need to be removed unless there is discomfort/pain or removal is requested. If the implant cannot be identified within the arm a chest X-ray should be undertaken.

- ◦ If removal is requested or the implant needs to be changed, refer to the regional centre providing deep implant removals.
- ◦ High resolution ultrasound will be used to locate the implant and it is normally removed through a small incision.
- ◦ If the implant cannot be located the manufacturer can arrange an etonogestrel assay in the Netherlands.
- Implants are flexible and can be bent or fractured by women, without apparently affecting their efficacy; they can remain *in situ*.

7.6.5 Advice about late removal of implants

Nexplanon is licensed to provide contraception for 3 years. If it is changed within the 3-year period no abstinence from sex or additional contraceptive method is required.

If more than 3 years has elapsed the chance of pregnancy is small. A pregnancy test should be performed and if negative, the implant can be changed with advice to use condoms for the next week. A pregnancy test should be repeated in a further 3 weeks. It is unlikely that emergency contraception will be needed if unprotected sex has occurred and the implant was fitted less than 4 years ago.

7.7 Routine follow-up

If the implant has been fitted following the 'quick-start' guidance (see *Table 7.1* and *Chapter 2*) a pregnancy test should be performed in 3 weeks. There is no need for a routine review; however, women should be advised to re-attend if:
- they have any concerns
- the implant needs to be changed
- the implant cannot be felt
- there is pain or irritation over the implant
- there are signs of infection or the implant appears broken.

7.8 Return to fertility

Following implant removal there is an immediate return to a woman's pre-existing fertility, with etonogestrel levels undetectable at 1 week. Most women start to ovulate within 3 weeks of implant removal.

7.9 Managing troublesome side-effects

7.9.1 Bleeding problems

- Take a careful medical and relationship history.
- Exclude STIs and any gynaecology pathology.
- Check, where applicable, that cervical screening is up-to-date.

- Perform a pelvic examination if there are other symptoms including dysmenorrhoea, dyspareunia, vaginal discharge, dysuria.
- Perform a pelvic examination if unexplained troublesome bleeding has persisted for more than 3 months or a medical treatment has failed to stop a bleeding episode. Treatment options to stop a bleeding episode include:
  - using a continuous or cyclical combined hormonal contraceptive (pill, patch or ring) for 3 months (outside of the product licence); this approach can be continued for longer if bleeding is controlled and the patient wishes to use the implant for contraception and the COC to control the bleeding
  - tranexamic acid 250 mg four a day for 5 days
  - mefenamic acid 500 mg up to 3 times a day for 5 days
  - anecdotally, one desogestrel POP daily or therapeutic doses of progestogen for up to 3 months (medroxyprogesterone acetate 10 mg up to 3 times a day continuously or for 21 days with a 7 day break).
- There is no evidence that these treatments confer a long-term benefit.

7.9.2 Headaches

Headaches are commonly reported by the general population with no causal link to implant use found. Suggest paracetamol/ibuprofen as appropriate.

7.9.3 Acne

Women switching from combined hormonal contraceptives to progestogen-only methods, such as implants, may complain of acne as sex hormone binding globulin levels fall and resultant free testosterone levels rise. Studies have shown that acne may improve, worsen or remain the same in implant users. Standard topical acne therapies can be tried.

7.10 Myths and misconceptions

- **Implants make you fat** – there is no evidence that implant users gain any more weight than their peers.
- **Implants are difficult to remove** – if they are fitted correctly in the subdermal plane, removal should be straightforward.
- **Implants make you bleed all the time** – most women are satisfied with their bleeding pattern, but the key is to give a realistic picture before fitting the implant. Unfortunately, some may assume they will have very little bleeding if their friends with implants have infrequent periods.

EXAMPLE

A 20 year old secretary has just had her implant changed and feels that she has more bloating with the new implant. She has also found that her menstrual bleeding pattern has changed as she is having more infrequent bleeds.

What do you advise?

1. Take a medical and relationship history.
2. Check when she had her implant changed.
3. Perform a pregnancy test and STI screen.
4. If all is fine, remind the patient that a new implant releases 50% more hormone when compared to her previous implant that had been in place for 3 years, which explains why she has noticed a change in her bleeding pattern. The bloating should improve over the first few months but she is likely to continue with infrequent periods.

References

British National Formulary, March 2023–September 2023.

eMC: SPC Nexplanon 68 mg implant for subdermal use [www.medicines.org.uk/emc/product/5720/smpc – accessed May 2023]

FSRH (2015) *Problematic Bleeding with Hormonal Contraception*. Clinical Effectiveness Unit. [www.fsrh.org/documents/ceuguidanceproblematicbleedinghormonalcontraception – accessed May 2023]

FSRH (2019) *Overweight, Obesity and Contraception*. Clinical Effectiveness Unit. [www.fsrh.org/standards-and-guidance/documents/fsrh-clinical-guideline-overweight-obesity-and-contraception – accessed May 2023]

FSRH (2021) *Progestogen-only Implants*. Clinical Effectiveness Unit. [www.fsrh.org/standards-and-guidance/fsrh-guidelines-and-statements/method-specific/progestogen-only-implants – accessed May 2023]

Office for National Statistics (2009) Opinions Survey Report No. 41 *Contraception and Sexual Health*, 2008/09.

UKMEC (2016) *UK Medical Eligibility Criteria for Contraceptive Use* [www.fsrh.org/ukmec – accessed May 2023]

Chapter 8
Intrauterine system

Intrauterine contraception (IUC) includes intrauterine systems (IUS) and intrauterine devices (IUD). IUCs provide cost-effective, reliable, long-acting and reversible contraception. While an IUS containing 52 mg levonorgestrel may be more suitable for women who have heavy bleeding, for those seeking an effective but non-hormonal method an IUD may be most appropriate. However, in many cases either an IUS or an IUD will be a suitable option for women to consider.

For simplicity and ease of access to information the IUS will be discussed in this chapter and the IUD in *Chapter 9*, although many of the issues discussed are applicable to all IUC methods.

There are four levonorgestrel-containing intrauterine systems (IUS) available in the UK. The first two contain 52 mg of levonorgestrel (IUS-52 – Mirena, Levosert and Benilexa). Mirena has been available in the UK since May 1995 and Levosert since April 2015. The third, containing 13.5 mg of levonorgestrel (IUS-13.5 – Jaydess), was launched in April 2014, and most recently Kyleena, with 19.5 mg of levonorgestrel (IUS-19.5), could be fitted from 2018. The 52 mg IUS is licensed for the treatment of heavy menstrual bleeding; recent FSRH guidance states that any IUS-52 can be used as the progestogen component of hormone replacement therapy.

8.1 Potential users

8.1.1 Most appropriate users

- For the majority of women the benefits of the IUS outweigh the risks.
- The IUS is suitable for all women of reproductive age until contraception is no longer required, providing there are no contraindications (see UKMEC in *Appendix*).
- An IUS can be used in women who have not had a previous pregnancy and continuation rates are similar for parous and nulliparous women.
- As the IUS provides immediately reversible contraception, it is well suited to women wishing to space pregnancies.
- An IUS offers long-term effective contraception and is a suitable alternative to sterilization for women who have completed their families.
- An IUS is the first-line medical treatment for heavy menstrual bleeding and will reduce dysmenorrhoea.
- An IUS can be used for women with undetectable β-hCG and a history of trophoblastic disease.

8.1.2 Not suitable for the following users

The IUS is not suitable for women with:
- unexplained vaginal bleeding
- post-partum women between 48 hours and 4 weeks post-delivery
- post-partum or post-abortion sepsis
- persistently elevated β-hCG or malignant gestational trophoblastic disease
- cervical cancer awaiting treatment
- endometrial cancer

- current pelvic inflammatory disease
- current chlamydia or gonorrhoea (unless the infection is asymptomatic and treatment is given. Decision whether or not to fit should be made on a case-by-case basis)
- known pelvic tuberculosis
- known serious cardiac conditions or arrhythmias where a vasovagal collapse may have serious consequences (see *Section 3.5*)
- HIV positive with a CD4 count <200 cells/mm^3.

8.2 Available intrauterine systems in the UK

These are detailed in *Table 8.1*.

Table 8.1 IUS available in the UK

Trade name	Hormonal content	Size of device	Duration of use	Cost
Benilexa	52 mg (initial release 20.1 micrograms/24h, release at end of licence 8.6 micrograms/24h)	32 × 32 mm Diameter of insertion tube – 4.8 mm One-handed inserter	6 years	£88.00 Drug tariff and £71.00 NHS indicative price
Levosert	52 mg (initial release 20.1 micrograms/24h, release at end of licence 8.6 micrograms/24h)	32 × 32 mm Diameter of insertion tube – 4.8 mm Two-handed inserter	6 years	£66.00 Drug tariff and £88.00 NHS indicative price
Mirena	52 mg (initial release 20 micrograms/24h, release at end of licence 9 micrograms/24h)	32 × 32 mm Diameter of insertion tube – 4.4 mm One-handed inserter	5 years	£88.00 Drug tariff and NHS indicative price
Kyleena	19.5 mg (initial release 17.5 micrograms/24h, release at end of licence 7.4 micrograms/24h	28 × 30 mm Diameter of insertion tube – 3.8 mm One-handed inserter	5 years	£76.00 Drug tariff and NHS indicative price
Jaydess	13.5 mg (initial release 14 micrograms/24h, release at end of licence 5 micrograms/24h	28 × 30 mm Diameter of insertion tube – 3.8 mm One-handed inserter	3 years	£69.22 Drug tariff and NHS indicative price

Data from FSRH, 2023 and *BNF*, 2023.

8.3 Mechanism of action

- The IUS exerts its main contraceptive action pre-fertilization by altering the cervical mucus and utero-tubal fluid, which inhibits sperm penetration and migration.
- The IUS down-regulates oestrogen and progesterone receptors within the endometrium, making it relatively insensitive to circulating oestrogen. This prevents endometrial proliferation causing atrophic changes to occur within a month of insertion. This will prevent implantation if fertilization occurs.
- The progestogen may affect sperm motility and function, preventing fertilization.

- Ovulation may be suppressed in a small number of users in the first year, possibly by reducing the pre-ovulatory LH surge. However, serum oestradiol levels are not reduced.

8.4 Efficacy

- The IUS-52 has a failure rate of up to 2 in 1000 over 5 years, with cumulative pregnancy rates of less than 1% at 5 years.
- The IUS-13.5 and IUS-19.5 have a similar failure rate of between 0.2% and 0.33% at 1 year with a cumulative failure rate of 0.9% at 3 years and 1.4% at 5 years, respectively.

8.5 Pros and cons of IUS

8.5.1 Advantages

- Long-acting and independent of sexual intercourse.
- Not affected by liver enzyme inducing drugs.
- Highly effective contraceptive (IUS-52 as effective as female sterilization) with an immediate return to fertility after removal. Increasing use of LARCs such as the IUS has led to a fall in requests for female sterilization in the UK.
- IUS-52 reduces menstrual blood loss in women with no period problems. About one-quarter of women will be amenorrhoeic by year 3 when using the IUS-52.
- IUS-52 reduces heavy menstrual bleeding by about 97% after 12 months, with an associated improvement in haemoglobin and serum ferritin; this has led to gynaecologists performing fewer hysterectomies in the UK. It can be used in women with coagulation disorders or taking anticoagulants.
- Long-term use may prevent fibroid formation.
- IUS-52 reduces heavy menstrual bleeding associated with the presence of fibroids and adenomyosis.
- IUS-52 reduces the incidence of dysmenorrhoea in the general population and for women with adenomyosis.
- IUS-52 may be a useful medical treatment for women suffering from endometriosis, with significant improvements in severity and frequency of pain/menstrual symptoms. It is also a good maintenance therapy following conservative surgery for endometriosis.
- No evidence that the IUS affects serum oestradiol levels and BMD.
- Reduces the risk of ectopic pregnancy and can be used in women with a past history of extra-uterine pregnancies.
- Reduces the incidence of pelvic inflammatory disease.
- Mirena (IUS-52) is licensed to be used as the progestogenic component of hormone replacement therapy.
- May protect against the development of endometrial hyperplasia. The IUS-52 (Mirena) has been shown to resolve endometrial hyperplasia without atypia in 92% of cases and endometrial hyperplasia with atypia in 67% of women. It should not be used in women with early endometrial cancer.
- Has a high user acceptance rate with 3 year continuation rates over 70%.

8.5.2 Disadvantages

- Can cause irregular/prolonged bleeding in the first 3 months in women using the IUS for contraception. Prolonged bleeding/spotting (6 months or more following fitting) may occur in those with heavy menstrual bleeding with or without fibroids. Pre-insertion counselling is important and a realistic picture, describing this menstrual disturbance, must be given.
- The IUS may be expelled or displaced in about 4–6% of cases, particularly if intra-cavity fibroids are present or in women complaining of heavy menstrual loss.
- The fitting may be painful.
- Failure to fit the IUS can occur in 1–2% of cases as a result of pain during insertion or difficulties passing the sound or device through the cervix. This may be due to an anatomical anomaly or operator technique. An alternative appointment with another more experienced fitter should be offered. An alternative contraceptive method should be provided in the interim.
- IUS use is associated with a small increased risk of pelvic infection immediately after fitting. The risk is increased 6-fold within the first 20 days following IUS insertion (1.6 per 1000 women-years). After day 20 the infection risk is low and remains low. The overall risk of PID is <1 in 100 in low-risk women.
- A small number of women may develop functional ovarian cysts, which tend to resolve over 6 months or so and rarely require surgical intervention. Often they are asymptomatic and are more common in users of IUS-52 than IUS-13.5 or IUS-19.5.
- Between 1% and 2% of IUS/IUD users may have non-visible threads requiring investigation such as a transvaginal ultrasound scan to confirm the IUC is located in the uterine cavity. They require referral to a specialist for removal.
- Rare complications such as perforation of the uterus/cervix may occur (less than 2 per 1000 devices fitted) but this is more common in breastfeeding women.
- Some progestogenic symptoms may occur in the first few months following fitting, such as breast tenderness, bloating or acne. These symptoms tend to improve with time.
- In the event of IUS failure, between 25% and 50% of pregnancies will be ectopic, although the overall risk of ectopic pregnancy is lower than in the general population. The ectopic rate for the IUS-52 is 0.02 per 100 women-years; 0.11 per 100 women-years for the IUS-13.5; and 0.2 per 100 women-years for the IUS-19.5.
- The IUS cannot be used as an emergency form of contraception.

8.6 Counselling

- A medical history should be taken to ensure medical eligibility, along with comprehensive counselling encompassing the advantages, disadvantages, side-effects, risks and details of the fitting procedure.
- Effective counselling helps women to choose the most appropriate contraceptive method.
- Women should be advised to abstain from sex following a normal period or use a bridging method until the IUS can be fitted.

- Take a sexual health history and undertake an STI screen (chlamydia screening as a minimum) in women under 25 years old, or in women older than 25 with a new partner or more than 1 partner in the preceding 12 months. The IUS can be fitted on the same day as counselling and STI screening in asymptomatic women who are not at risk of pregnancy.
- There is no need to screen for bacterial vaginosis or candida infections.
- If the IUS is being used for heavy menstrual bleeding or dysmenorrhoea, further investigation such as full blood count, ultrasound scan and endometrial biopsy may be indicated.
- Women should be advised to seek help if they have heavy bleeding or severe pain after the IUS is fitted, if they develop an abnormal smelly vaginal discharge or if they think they are pregnant. If a pregnancy is confirmed by a urinary/serum pregnancy test then its site should be ascertained by ultrasound scan.
- Provide written information about the method, such as the Family Planning Association leaflet, available at www.fpa.org.uk/sites/default/files/ius-your-guide.pdf.
- *Table 8.2* provides a summary of topics to be included during discussion and in written information.

Table 8.2 Topics to cover during counselling and in written information

Topics
Advantages and disadvantages
Efficacy and mechanism of action
Perforation rate – up to 2 per 1000; this rate is increased 6-fold in breastfeeding women within 36 weeks of delivery (Heinemann *et al.*, 2015a)
Expulsion rate – 1 in 20; highest in the first 3 months post-insertion and during menstruation
Infection – 6-fold increased risk of PID in the first 20 days post-insertion, after which risk is low and remains low
Pregnancy and ectopic risk – pregnancy risk less than 1% a year and overall ectopic pregnancy risk very low, but if pregnancy occurs 25–50% may be ectopic
Bleeding pattern changes – at least 1 in 4 women using IUS-52 (this increases to 60% with a subsequent IUS); 1 in 19 women using IUS-19.5; and 1 in 13 women using IUS-13.5 experience amenorrhoea after 36 months
Hormonal side-effects – more common in the first few months of use and decrease over time; these include breast tenderness, headaches, acne and mood changes
Bridging contraception until the IUS is fitted – abstain or use effective method of contraception

8.7 IUS starting regimen

This is described in *Table 8.3*.

Table 8.3 Starting regimens for IUS

Circumstances	Start when?	Requirement for 7 days of additional contraceptive precautions?
Natural menstrual cycle	Up to and including day 7 (avoiding insertion when menstrual flow is heavy, to reduce chance of subsequent expulsion)	No
	After day 7 of the cycle, at any other time if it is reasonably certain she is not pregnant and/or a high sensitivity urine pregnancy test (HSUPT) is negative	Yes
Amenorrhoea	At any time if it is reasonably certain she is not pregnant and/or a HSUPT is negative	Yes
Quick starting	Should not generally be quick started unless pregnancy can be reasonably excluded	Not applicable
Following childbirth	Within the first 48 hours post-partum	No
	After day 28 (including following a caesarean section) providing the fitter is reasonably certain the woman is not pregnant	Yes unless inserted day 1–7 of cycle or LAM criteria are met
Following abortion, miscarriage, ectopic pregnancy or gestational trophoblastic disease	Within 7 days of the event	No
	After 7 days of the event	Yes
	IUS should not be inserted in women with persistently elevated hCG levels or malignant gestational trophoblastic disease	
Following emergency contraception	Should not be inserted following administration of oral EC until pregnancy can be excluded	Not applicable
Switching from a CHC	Day 1 of the HFI or week 2 or 3 of CHC cycle	No
	After day 1 of the HFI or in week 1 of CHC cycle	Continue CHC or use other additional contraception for 7 days
Switching from a traditional POP	At any time	Yes, continue POP or use additional contraception for 7 days
Switching from progestogen-only anovulatory methods		
• desogestrel pill	At any time	No
• injectable	Start any time up to when repeat injection is due	No
• implant	Start any time up to when implant is due for removal	No
Switching from IUD	Insert the IUS up to and including day 7 of a cycle	No
	After day 7, advise no sexual intercourse for 7 days prior to the IUS fitting	Yes

(continued)

Circumstances	Start when?	Requirement for 7 days of additional contraceptive precautions?
Switching IUS	If a woman is using an IUS in licence and is amenorrhoeic or has irregular bleeds, advise no sexual intercourse for 7 days prior to the changing of the IUS	No
	If insertion of IUS-52 occurred 6–7 years ago in a woman under age 45, removal and re-insertion may occur immediately if pregnancy test is negative, with a repeat pregnancy test no sooner than 3 weeks after last episode of UPSI	Yes
	If insertion of IUS-52 occurred >7 years ago in a woman under age 45, replacement should be delayed for at least 3 weeks after last UPSI and at which time a pregnancy test should be undertaken	Yes
	Women who retain their 13.5 mg LNG-IUS for more than 3 years should be advised to use additional precautions until pregnancy can be excluded, after which time a replacement device can be inserted	Yes
	If IUS-52 fitted in women at any age as the progestogen component of HRT, it will need changing every 5 years	
IUS in over 45-year-olds	If IUS-52 fitted in women of 45 years or older for contraception, it can remain in place until aged 55	Not applicable
	If IUS-52 fitted in women of 45 years or older for heavy menstrual bleeding only (for example she or her partner have been sterilized), it can remain in place as long as it is effective	

8.8 IUS insertion

- Undertake a bimanual examination to assess the size, position, shape and motility of the uterus and exclude pathology.
- Using a non-touch (aseptic) technique insert a speculum, hold cervix with forceps (Allis or tenaculum) and apply gentle traction to straighten uterine flexion and reduce the risk of perforation.
- Assess cavity length with a uterine sound.
- Insert the IUS following the product recommendations, ensuring final placement is at the fundus of the uterus. Each product has a slightly different insertion technique, therefore it is important for fitters to be appropriately trained.
- Trim the threads so that they are 3–4 cm long outside the external os of the cervix.

8.9 Post IUS insertion advice

- Instructions are given on how and when to check the IUC threads, initially before they start having sex and then on a monthly basis.

- If the threads cannot be felt, additional contraception such as condoms should be used and an appointment made with the doctor or nurse in their GP surgery or at a local sexual health clinic.
- Post-insertion pain is common and can occur for up to a week following placement. If this does not resolve with simple analgesics women are advised to return for assessment.
- If there are symptoms suggestive of infection, such as foul-smelling discharge, abdominal pain and fever, assessment should be undertaken by a general practitioner or at a local sexual health clinic.

8.10 Routine follow-up

- Routine follow-up appointments after IUC fitting are no longer required as they have not been shown to be effective in detecting problems associated with placement.
- Women are advised to attend if they cannot feel the IUS threads or they appear longer, or they can feel the tip of the device. In all cases additional contraception should be used until they have been examined by a clinician.
- Advice should be sought if women develop severe abdominal pains, heavy menstrual bleeding or they have a positive pregnancy test, to exclude pelvic infection, mal-position of the IUS or an ectopic pregnancy.
- Women should seek help if they continue to experience problematic vaginal bleeding patterns after the first 3–6 months.

8.11 Return to fertility and device removal

- Following removal of the IUS there is no delay in return to fertility.
- To avoid an unplanned pregnancy the IUS should be removed when there has been no unprotected sex for the preceding 7 days.

8.12 Managing side-effects and complications

8.12.1 Spotting or bleeding

- Irregular, light or prolonged bleeding commonly occurs in IUS users, particularly in the first 3–6 months of use, and typically settles without treatment.
- Histologically large thin-walled blood vessels appear within an atrophic endometrium which may explain the unscheduled bleeding experienced by some users.
- If there are no contraindications, CHC can be used for 3 months either cyclically or continuously. Longer-term use is based on clinical judgement. Oral progestogens even in high dose are not effective.

8.12.2 Non-visible threads

- If previously palpable/visible threads become impalpable/non-visible there are three main issues to consider:

- ○ the threads may have been drawn up into the uterine cavity
  - ○ the device may have been expelled
  - ○ the device may have translocated into the abdominal cavity.
- If the threads cannot be felt, women are advised to use an alternative method of contraception until clinical assessment can be undertaken.
- At this assessment a pregnancy test is recommended.
  - ○ The endocervical canal can be gently explored; however, an ultrasound scan to confirm the presence of the IUS within the uterine cavity is the preferred approach. Once correct placement has been determined the IUS can remain *in situ* with no additional follow-up needed or, if removal is required, an IUS thread retriever or forceps should be used.
  - ○ If the ultrasound scan fails to locate the IUS then an abdominal X-ray is advised to exclude the presence of the device within the abdominal cavity before expulsion can be assumed.

8.12.3 Managing IUS insertion pain

- There is some evidence to support the use of naproxen 500 mg taken 1 hour before IUC fitting for pain management during insertion; NSAIDs are also effective in the management of post-insertion pain.
- Lidocaine 10% spray applying 4 puffs to the cervix and waiting 3 minutes is more effective than placebo for relieving insertion pain. 5% lidocaine/prilocaine cream placed on a cotton bud with 2 ml applied to the anterior cervical lip and 2 ml placed around the os may reduce pain as long as the fitter waits 7 minutes after application. Studies have shown that a paracervical/intracervical block may reduce pain, benefiting those who require cervical dilation or who are very anxious.
- There is currently no evidence to suggest a particular type of forceps used to stabilize the cervix is associated with reduced insertion pain.

8.12.4 Pregnancy associated with an IUS

- As amenorrhoea is common in IUS users, women with pregnancy symptoms and a positive pregnancy test should seek immediate medical advice.
- The site of the pregnancy should be confirmed by ultrasound scan, with suspected ectopic pregnancies managed as a gynaecological emergency.
- In women with an intrauterine pregnancy, the presence of an IUS in the uterine cavity increases the risk of early or mid-trimester pregnancy loss, sepsis and pre-term labour.
- If a woman presents before 12 weeks of pregnancy the device should be removed if the threads are visible but the uterus should not be instrumented.
- If the pregnancy is greater than 12 weeks the IUS should be left *in situ*. It is normally expelled with the placenta at delivery. If the IUS is not found at delivery then an abdominal X-ray should be performed to exclude translocation.
- There is currently no evidence that the presence of an IUS during pregnancy is associated with birth defects.

8.12.5 Actinomycosis-like organisms

- Actinomycosis-like organisms are normal commensals of the genital tract and their presence is not diagnostic of a disease process.
- Symptoms of pelvic actinomycosis including pain, dyspareunia, excessive discharge, and an adnexal mass.
  - in the absence of symptoms it is not necessary to remove the IUC
  - if symptoms are present, an IUS removal should be considered followed by antibiotics in accordance with local policy.

8.12.6 Syncope and bradycardia at insertion

- Bradycardia is a heart rate of <60 beats per minute, although symptoms do not typically occur until the heart rate reaches <40 beats per minute.
- Symptoms include feeling faint, dizziness and light-headedness, pallor, sweating, nausea and vomiting, and loss of consciousness which may be associated with twitching or a brief seizure.
- If associated with IUS insertions symptoms occur as a result of vagal stimulation following dilation of the internal cervical os or instrumentation of the uterus.
- Symptoms are generally transient and resolve as the bradycardia resolves.
- With regard to management, the procedure should be stopped and the foot of the examination couch raised. Pulse and blood pressure should be monitored and supplemental oxygen given at 10–15 L/min.
- If pulse is less than 40 beats per minute and the IUS is in the uterine cavity the device should be removed and atropine administered (500 micrograms IV or IM into the mid thigh). If there is no improvement after 5 mins call for emergency assistance or an ambulance. A further dose of atropine can be given after 5 mins for IV and 10 mins for IM administration.

8.12.7 IUS perforation

- If recognized at the time of the IUS fit, removal should be undertaken and arrangements made for re-fitting by a senior fitter in a month's time.
- If IUS perforation is identified at a later date, surgical removal by laparoscopy is advised.

8.12.8 Failure to insert an IUS

- The procedure is abandoned, bridging contraception provided and a follow-up appointment scheduled with a more experienced fitter.

8.12.9 Suspected pelvic infection

- If pelvic infection is clinically diagnosed and appropriate antibiotics are commenced, the IUS can be kept *in situ*. Current recommendations for the treatment of PID are:

- ◦ ceftriaxone 1 g intramuscularly single dose followed by
  oral doxycycline 100 mg twice daily plus
  metronidazole 400 mg twice daily for 14 days, OR
- ◦ oral ofloxacin 400 mg twice daily plus oral metronidazole 400 mg twice daily
  for 14 days; both regimens provide cover against chlamydia and gonorrhoea as
  well as aerobic and anaerobic organisms. See the British Association for Sexual
  Health and HIV (www.bashh.org) for further details.
- Only remove the IUS if symptoms fail to improve following 72 hours of antibiotic
  use.
- Ensure partner notification is undertaken and sexual health advice is provided.
- Advise the woman not to have sex until the infection has been treated and her
  partner has completed their course of appropriate antibiotics.

8.13 Myths and misconceptions

- **The IUS causes weight gain** – there is no evidence to suggest that the IUS causes
  additional weight gain. Unfortunately women gain weight over time.
- **There is good evidence that the IUS reduces your sex drive** – there is
  contradictory evidence about an association between libido and the use of
  hormonal contraception. Better studies are required where users are not aware of
  the contraceptive method used.
- **An IUS can only be used by women who have had children** – the IUS is suitable
  for all women of reproductive age whether they have had children or not.
- **Women who are taking anticoagulants cannot have an IUS fitted** – this is not
  true; in fact an IUS may reduce menstrual blood loss associated with the use of this
  medication.

EXAMPLE

**A 32 year old woman attends for an IUS fitting. She is in a new relationship and
was therefore offered an STI screen prior to her IUS fit. She is positive for genital
chlamydia but is asymptomatic. She wants the IUS to be fitted immediately.**

What do you do?

1. Confirm infection is asymptomatic.
2. Following counselling about the possible risks, an IUS could be inserted in an
   asymptomatic woman who has completed antibiotic treatment or on the day that
   treatment is commenced.
3. If the results of an infection screen are not available at the time of IUS fitting, the
   IUS should still be inserted without antibiotic prophylaxis, providing the woman is
   asymptomatic, contactable and willing to return for treatment if necessary.
4. In women with symptoms of possible or confirmed infection, IUS insertion should
   be delayed until the infection is treated and symptoms have resolved and a
   bridging method provided.

References

British Association for Sexual Health and HIV (2019) *UK National Guideline for the Management of Pelvic Inflammatory Disease*. Clinical Effectiveness Group. [www.bashhguidelines.org/current-guidelines/systemic-presentation-and-complications/pid-2019/ – accessed May 2023]

British National Formulary, March 2023–September 2023.

FSRH (2021) *Statement: Pain associated with insertion of intrauterine contraception*. [www.fsrh.org/standards-and-guidance/documents/fsrh-statement-pain-associated-with-insertion-of-intrauterine – accessed May 2023]

FSRH (2022) *Service Standards for Resuscitation in Sexual and Reproductive Healthcare Services*. [www.fsrh.org/documents/fsrh-service-standards-for-resuscitation – accessed May 2023]

FSRH (2023) *Clinical Guideline: intrauterine contraception*. Clinical Effectiveness Unit. [www.fsrh.org/standards-and-guidance/fsrh-guidelines-and-statements/method-specific/intrauterine-contaception – accessed May 2023]

Heinemann, K. *et al.* (2015a) Risk of uterine perforation with levonorgestrel-releasing and copper intrauterine devices in the European Active Surveillance Study on Intrauterine Devices. *Contraception*, **91**: 274–279.

Heinemann, K. *et al.* (2015b) Comparative contraceptive effectiveness of levonorgestrel-releasing and copper intrauterine devices: the European Active Surveillance Study for Intrauterine Devices. *Contraception*, **91**: 280–283.

Office for National Statistics (2009) Opinions Survey Report No. 41 *Contraception and Sexual Health*, 2008/09.

UKMEC (2016) *UK Medical Eligibility Criteria for Contraceptive Use* [www.fsrh.org/ukmec – accessed May 2023]

Chapter 9
Copper intrauterine devices

Over 180 million women worldwide use IUDs, with nearly 50% of these users in China. In the UK, only 6% of women use this form of contraception, probably because of concerns and myths attached to this method. The available IUDs in the UK are small copper-containing devices with most having a central frame made of polyethylene impregnated with barium sulphate to make them radiopaque. They come in varying shapes and sizes, including a frameless device called a GyneFix and an intrauterine ball called Ballerine. Most devices contain more than 300 mm^2 of copper, making them a highly effective, reversible, inexpensive contraceptive option for women.

9.1 Potential users

9.1.1 Most appropriate users

- IUDs are an ideal choice for women who request a reliable non-hormonal method of contraception.
- The IUD is suitable for women until contraception is no longer required, providing there are no contraindications.
- An IUD can be used in women who have not had a previous pregnancy and continuation rates are similar for parous and nulliparous women.
- As the IUD provides immediately reversible contraception, it is well suited to women wishing to space pregnancies.
- An IUD offers long-term effective contraception and so it provides a suitable alternative to sterilization for women who have completed their families.
- An IUD may be used as a method of emergency contraception (see *Chapter 13*).
- An IUD can be used for women with undetectable β-hCG and a history of trophoblastic disease.

9.1.2 Not suitable for the following users

The IUD is not suitable for women:
- with unexplained vaginal bleeding
- with post-partum and post-abortion sepsis
- post-partum between 48 hours and 4 weeks post-delivery
- with persistently elevated β-hCG or malignant gestational trophoblastic disease
- with cervical cancer awaiting treatment
- with endometrial cancer
- with current pelvic inflammatory disease
- with current chlamydia or gonorrhoea (unless the infection is asymptomatic and treatment is given; the decision whether or not to fit should be made on a case-by-case basis)
- with known pelvic tuberculosis
- with known serious cardiac conditions or arrhythmias where a vasovagal collapse may have serious consequences (see *Section 3.5*)
- HIV positive with a CD4 count <200 cells/mm^3.

9.2 Available IUDs in the UK

Details of the range of IUDs available in the UK are provided in *Table 9.1*.

Table 9.1 IUDs available in the UK

Trade name	Copper content	Location of copper	Cavity length	Duration of use	Cost
Ancora 375 Cu	375 mm^2	Vertical stem	>6.5 cm	5 years	£7.95
Copper T 380A	380 mm^2	Vertical stem and copper sleeve on each arm	6.5–9 cm	10 years	£8.95
Flexi-T 300	300 mm^2	Vertical stem	>5 cm	5 years	£9.47
Flexi-T + 380	380 mm^2	Vertical stem and copper sleeve on each arm	>6 cm	5 years	£10.06
GyneFix	330 mm^2	6 copper sleeves on polypropylene thread	Any size	5 years	£27.11
Load 375	375 mm^2	Vertical stem	>7 cm	5 years	£8.52
Mini TT 380 Slimline	380 mm^2	Vertical stem and copper sleeves fitted flush on to distal portion of each horizontal arm	>5 cm	5 years	£12.46
Multiload Cu375	375 mm^2	Vertical stem	6–9 cm	5 years	£9.24
Multi-Safe 375	375 mm^2	Vertical stem	6–9 cm	5 years	£8.96
Neo-Safe T380	380 mm^2	Vertical stem	6.5–9 cm	5 years	£13.40
Novaplus T 380 Ag	380 mm^2	Vertical stem	Mini is 5 cm and normal size is 6.5–9 cm	5 years	£12.50
Novaplus T 380 Cu	380 mm^2	Vertical stem	Mini is 5 cm and normal size is 6.5–9 cm	5 years	£10.95
Nova-T 380	380 mm^2	Vertical stem	6.5–9 cm	5 years	£15.20
T-Safe 380A QuickLoad	380 mm^2	Vertical stem with copper collar on the distal portion of each arm	6.5–9 cm	10 years	£10.55
TT 380 Slimline	380 mm^2	Vertical stem, and copper sleeves fitted flush on to distal portion of each horizontal arm	6.5–9 cm	10 years	£12.46

(continued)

Trade name	Copper content	Location of copper	Cavity length	Duration of use	Cost
UT 380 Short	380 mm²	Vertical stem	5–7 cm	5 years	£11.22
UT 380 Standard	380 mm²	Vertical stem	6.5–9 cm	5 years	£11.22

Data from *BNF*, 2023.

9.3 Mechanism of action

- The main mechanism of action is to prevent fertilization through a foreign body effect and the copper ion's toxicity to sperm and ova.
- All IUDs increase the number of leukocytes in the endometrium. This produces a 'sterile' inflammatory endometrial response helping to prevent implantation. This reaction is enhanced by copper. Copper also affects endothelial enzymes, glycogen metabolism and oestrogen uptake.
- Copper content of the cervico-uterine mucus is high and this inhibits sperm penetration.
- An IUD is not an abortifacient because medicolegally, pregnancy begins at implantation not fertilization.

9.4 Efficacy

- Overall this method is associated with a failure rate of around 2% after 10 years and 0.1–1% after the first year of use. This equates to a failure rate of up to 2 in 1000 over 5 years.
- FSRH (2015) recommend the use of T-shaped IUDs containing 380 mm² of copper with banded copper on the arms of the device.

9.5 Pros and cons of IUDs

9.5.1 Advantages

- Long-term (up to 10 years depending on the device fitted), highly effective contraception, with no delay in return to fertility following removal.
- Non-hormonal contraceptive method, therefore no hormonal side-effects.
- Effective immediately after fitting.
- Non-intercourse related method of contraception.
- Efficacy is not affected by liver enzyme inducing medication.
- Can be used when breastfeeding.
- Very low morbidity, with a mortality rate of less than 1 per 500 000 users.
- The most effective method of emergency contraception:
  - can be fitted up to 5 days after unprotected sexual intercourse at any time in the cycle

- ○ can also be fitted up to 5 days following the earliest estimated time of ovulation, even if multiple episodes of unprotected sex have occurred.
- High acceptability with first year continuation rates of almost 80%. IUDs are ideal for nulliparous women, those spacing their children or those whose family is complete.
- Inexpensive and very cost-effective contraceptive method.
- Highly effective method of contraception.
- May give up to 50% protection against the development of endometrial cancer.

9.5.2 Disadvantages

- May cause menstrual irregularities, with intermenstrual bleeding and spotting occurring more commonly within the first 6 months after IUD insertion.
- Pain or discomfort may be experienced for a few hours to up to a week following insertion.
- Failure to fit the IUD – although uncommon, failure may occur as a result of pain during insertion, anxiety or difficulties passing the uterine sound or device through the cervix; this may be due to anatomical anomaly or operator technique. The woman should be offered an alternative appointment with a more experienced fitter, with care taken to provide an alternative method of contraception in the interim.
- Periods **may** become heavier, more prolonged and more painful. Periods may last 1–2 days longer, with blood loss increasing by about one-third. There may be more pre-/post-menstrual spotting and dysmenorrhoea. Intermenstrual bleeding and spotting is common in the first 3–6 months of IUD use. About 10% of women will discontinue using an IUD in the first year citing menstrual bleeding +/– pain as the main reason for removal. These problems may be managed with analgesics.
- IUDs provide no protection against STIs.
- About 1 in 20 IUDs are expelled, with this more likely to occur within the first 3 months after fitting, and the rate is similar for all types of IUD. Expulsion can lead to an unplanned pregnancy.
- IUD use is associated with a small increased risk of pelvic infection immediately after fitting. The risk is increased 6-fold within the first 20 days following IUD insertion (1.6 per 1000 women-years). After day 20 the infection risk is low and remains low. The overall risk of PID is <1 in 100 in low-risk women.
- Uterine perforation is an uncommon event and may occur in up to 2 per 1000 insertions. Different IUDs are not associated with an increased or decreased risk of perforation, but the risk is increased 6-fold in women who are breastfeeding. Perforation rates are influenced by fitter experience and the risk is higher in first-time users compared to previous users.
- IUDs are associated with a low risk of pregnancy. However, if pregnancy does occur approximately 15% will be ectopic. The incidence of ectopic pregnancy in IUD users is 0.08 per 100 women-years compared to 1.1 per 100 in UK women not using any contraception each year. Therefore, while the absolute risk of an ectopic pregnancy is lower in users of IUDs when compared to a background population, if a pregnancy does occur approximately 1 in 6 will be ectopic.

9.6 Counselling

- A medical history should be undertaken to ensure medical eligibility. Prior to fitting, comprehensive counselling encompassing the advantages, disadvantages, side-effects, risks and details of the fitting procedure is recommended.
- Effective counselling helps ensure patient satisfaction and longevity of method use.
- STI history and screening (chlamydia screening as a minimum) is recommended prior to IUD insertion in women under 25 years old, or in women older than 25 with a new partner or more than 1 partner in the preceding 12 months. In asymptomatic women attending for insertion of an IUD there is no need to delay the fitting until results of a screen are available, providing that a screen has been or is taken at the time of fitting and the woman will return for treatment if required. If the IUD is fitted as an emergency, prophylactic treatment for chlamydia +/− gonorrhoea may be considered for women who are symptomatic or at high risk of infection.
- There is no need to routinely screen for bacterial vaginosis or candida infection.
- Pregnancy should be excluded prior to IUD insertion. Therefore, advise no sex following their period or provide a bridging method or fit as emergency contraception (see *Chapter 13*).
- Advise women to seek help urgently if they are concerned that they might be pregnant in order to perform a pregnancy test and, if positive, arrange an urgent ultrasound scan to locate the site of the pregnancy.
- Provide written information about the method, such as the Family Planning Association leaflet (available at www.sexwise.fpa.org.uk).
- See *Table 9.2* for a summary of topics to be included during the discussion and in written information.

Table 9.2 Topics to include during counselling and in written information

Topics
Advantages and disadvantages
Efficacy and mechanism of action
Perforation rate – up to 2 per 1000; the rate is increased 6-fold in breastfeeding women less than 36 weeks since delivery (Heinemann *et al.*, 2015a)
Expulsion rate – 1 in 20, highest in the first 3 months post-insertion and during menstruation
Infection – 6-fold increased risk of PID in the first 20 days post-insertion, after which risk is low and remains low
Pregnancy and ectopic risk – pregnancy risk is 2 in 1000 over 5 years and ectopic risk was recently reported as 0.08 per 100 women-years (Heinemann *et al.*, 2015b)
Bleeding pattern – intermenstrual spotting is common for 3–6 months post-insertion; pre- and post-menstrual spotting is common and periods are often more painful
Contraception until fitting – abstain or continue current method of contraception

9.7 IUD starting regimen

This is described in *Table 9.3* below.

Table 9.3 Starting regimens for IUDs

Circumstances	Start when?	Requirement for 7 days of additional contraceptive precautions?
Natural menstrual cycle	At any time if it is reasonably certain she is not pregnant and/or a high sensitivity urine pregnancy test (HSUPT) is negative	No
Amenorrhoea	At any time if it is reasonably certain she is not pregnant and/or a HSUPT is negative	No
Quick starting	Only if the indications for EC are met (see *Chapter 13*)	
Following childbirth	Within the first 48 hours post-partum	No
	After day 28 (including following a caesarean section) providing the fitter is reasonably certain the woman is not pregnant	No
Following abortion, miscarriage, ectopic pregnancy or gestational trophoblastic disease	Immediately	No
	At any time by an experienced clinician as long as there is no concern that the pregnancy is ongoing	No
	IUC should not be inserted in women with persistently elevated hCG levels or malignant gestational trophoblastic disease	
Following emergency contraception	Outside of the criteria for insertion of a Cu-IUD for EC an IUD should not be inserted following administration of oral EC until pregnancy can be excluded by a pregnancy test no sooner than 3 weeks after the last episode of UPSI	
Switching from hormonal methods • COC • traditional POP • desogestrel pill • injectable • implant	Inserted at any time if another method of contraception has been used consistently and correctly and it is reasonably certain that the woman is not pregnant or at risk of pregnancy	No
Switching from LNG-IUS	Ideally if switching from an LNG-IUS to a Cu-IUD additional contraceptive precautions are advised in the 7 days before changing in case the new method cannot be inserted	No
Switching IUD	Women who wish replacement of a Cu-IUD outside the licensed duration of use should have pregnancy reliably excluded prior to the replacement	No

9.8 IUD insertion

- Undertake a bimanual examination to assess the size, position, shape and motility of the uterus and to exclude pathology.
- Using a non-touch (aseptic) technique insert a speculum and then apply forceps (Allis or tenaculum) to the cervix to stabilize it and reduce the risk of perforation.
- Assess cavity length with a uterine sound.
- Insert the IUD as per the product recommendations, ensuring that devices are placed at the fundus.
- Trim the threads to approximately 3–4 cm long outside the external os of the cervix.

9.9 Post IUD insertion advice

- Rest for a few minutes following the fitting.
- Instructions should be given on how and when to check IUD threads (initially prior to having sex following the fit, and then on a monthly basis) and when to seek advice; for example, if the threads feel longer than normal, if the woman is unable to feel the threads, or if the tip of the device is felt.
- Post-insertion pain is common in the first few days up to a week after insertion; however, if this is not resolved with simple analgesics individuals are advised to return for assessment.
- If there are symptoms suggestive of infection, such as foul-smelling discharge, abdominal pain and fever, medical assessment is recommended.

9.10 Routine follow-up

- Routine follow-up appointments after IUC fitting are no longer required as they have not been shown to be effective in detecting problems associated with placement.
- Women are advised to attend if they cannot feel the IUC threads or they appear longer, or they can feel the tip of the device. In all cases additional contraception should be used until they have been examined by a clinician.
- Advice should be sought if women develop severe abdominal pains, heavy menstrual bleeding or they have a positive pregnancy test, in order to exclude pelvic infection, mal-position of the IUC or an ectopic pregnancy.
- Women should seek help if they continue to experience problematic vaginal bleeding patterns after the first 3–6 months.

9.11 Return to fertility and device removal

- When an IUD is removed there is no delay in return to fertility because the hormonal cycle is not altered.
- The device can be removed at any time in the cycle. If the woman does not wish to risk becoming pregnant immediately then she should be advised to abstain or use condoms for the 7 days preceding removal.

9.12 Managing side-effects and complications

9.12.1 Spotting or bleeding

- Spotting or light bleeding is commonly experienced during the first 3–6 months of IUD use, but it usually decreases with time.
- If bleeding continues or is heavy and prolonged a careful history and examination should be undertaken, plus additional investigations to exclude STIs, pregnancy and gynaecological pathology, as appropriate.
- An antifibrinolytic such as tranexamic acid 1 g taken 3 times a day can be used on days 1–4 of bleeding +/– an NSAID (ibuprofen 400 mg 3 times a day or mefenamic acid 500 mg 3 times a day).
- If heavy bleeding is unacceptable or causes anaemia, discuss changing the contraceptive method to an IUS or an alternative LARC.

9.12.2 Vaginal discharge

- An increased watery or mucoid discharge is common in IUD users; if this becomes profuse, persistent or offensive it is important to rule out infection.
- Bacterial vaginosis has been found in some studies to be more common among IUD users than among non-IUD users. However, recent studies indicate that it is the irregular bleeding rather than the presence of the IUD that is associated with bacterial vaginosis.

9.12.3 Non-visible threads

- If previously palpable/visible threads become impalpable/non-visible there are three main issues to consider:
  - the threads may have been drawn up into the uterine cavity
  - the device has been expelled
  - the device has translocated into the abdominal cavity.
- If the threads cannot be felt, women are advised to use an alternative method of contraception until clinical assessment can be undertaken.
- At this assessment a pregnancy test is recommended.
  - The endocervical canal can be gently explored; however, an ultrasound scan to confirm the presence of the IUD within the uterine cavity is the preferred approach. Once correct placement has been determined, the IUD can remain *in situ* or, if removal is required, an IUD thread retriever or removal forceps should be used.
  - If the ultrasound scan fails to locate the IUD then an abdominal X-ray is advised to exclude the presence of the device within the abdominal cavity before expulsion can be assumed.

9.12.4 Managing IUD insertion pain

- There is some evidence to support the use of naproxen 500 mg taken 1 hour before IUC fitting for pain management during insertion; NSAIDs are also effective in the management of post-insertion pain.
- Lidocaine 10% spray applying 4 puffs to the cervix and waiting 3 minutes is more effective than placebo for relieving insertion pain. 5% lidocaine/prilocaine cream placed on a cotton bud with 2 ml applied to the anterior cervical lip and 2 ml placed around the os may reduce pain as long as the fitter waits 7 minutes after application. Studies have shown that a paracervical/intracervical block may reduce pain, benefiting those who require cervical dilation or who are very anxious.
- There is currently no evidence to suggest a particular type of forceps used to stabilize the cervix is associated with reduced insertion pain.

9.12.5 Pregnancy with an IUD *in utero*

- Women should seek urgent advice if they have a late or missed period. An ectopic pregnancy should be ruled out by performing an ultrasound scan to confirm the location of the pregnancy.
- In women with an intrauterine pregnancy, the presence of an IUD within the uterine cavity increases the risk of early or mid-trimester pregnancy loss, sepsis and pre-term labour.
- If a woman presents before 12 weeks of pregnancy the device should be removed if the threads are visible but the uterus should not be instrumented.
- If the pregnancy is greater than 12 weeks the IUD should be left *in situ*. It is normally expelled with the placenta at delivery. If the IUD is not found at delivery then an abdominal X-ray should be performed to exclude translocation.

9.12.6 Actinomycosis-like organisms

- Actinomycosis-like organisms are common commensals of the genital tract and their presence is not diagnostic of a disease process.
- Symptoms of pelvic actinomycosis include pain, dyspareunia, excessive discharge, and an adnexal mass:
  - in the absence of symptoms it is not necessary to remove the IUD
  - if symptoms are present, IUD removal should be considered followed by antibiotics in accordance with local policy.

9.12.7 Syncope and bradycardia at IUD insertion

- Bradycardia is a heart rate of <60 beats per minute, although symptoms do not typically occur until the heart rate reaches <40 beats per minute.
- Symptoms include feeling faint, dizziness and light-headedness, pallor, sweating, nausea and vomiting, and loss of consciousness which may be associated with twitching or a brief seizure.

- If associated with IUD insertion symptoms occur as a result of vagal stimulation following dilation of the internal cervical os or instrumentation of the uterus.
- Symptoms are generally transient and resolve as the bradycardia resolves.
- With regard to management, the procedure should be stopped and the foot of the examination couch raised. Pulse and blood pressure should be monitored and supplemental oxygen given at 10–15 L/min.
- If pulse is less than 40 beats per minute and the IUD is in the uterine cavity the device should be removed and atropine administered at 500 micrograms IV or IM into the mid thigh. If there is no improvement after 5 mins, call for emergency assistance or an ambulance. A further dose of atropine can be given after 5 min for IV and 10 min for IM administration.

9.12.8 IUD perforation

- If recognized at the time of IUD fit, removal should be undertaken and arrangements made for re-fitting by a senior fitter in a month's time.
- If IUD perforation is identified at a later date, surgical removal by laparoscopy is advisable because copper IUDs can cause an inflammatory reaction within the peritoneal cavity, leading to adhesions.

9.12.9 Failure to insert an IUD

- The procedure is abandoned, bridging contraception provided and a follow-up appointment made to re-attempt insertion.
- If re-attempt fails, either undertake a trial of insertion using a narrower device or refer to your local specialist.

9.12.10 Suspected pelvic infection

- If pelvic infection is clinically diagnosed and appropriate antibiotics are commenced, the IUD can be kept *in situ*. Current recommendations for the treatment of PID are:
  - ceftriaxone 1 g single dose followed by
    oral doxycycline 100 mg twice daily plus
    metronidazole 400 mg twice daily for 14 days, OR
  - oral ofloxacin 400 mg twice daily plus oral metronidazole 400 mg twice daily for 14 days, both of which provide cover against chlamydia and gonorrhoea, as well as aerobic and anaerobic organisms. See the British Association for Sexual Health and HIV (www.bashh.org) for further details.
- Only remove the IUD if symptoms fail to improve following 72 hours of antibiotic use.
- Ensure partner notification is undertaken and sexual health advice is provided.
- Advise the woman not to have sex until the infection has been treated and her partner has completed their course of appropriate antibiotics.

9.13 Myths and misconceptions

- **IUDs cause infection** – this is not true. Unprotected sex with a partner infected with an STI causes pelvic infection. Women using a copper IUD have no protection against the upper genital tract sequelae of STIs.
- **An IUD will cause scarring of the Fallopian tubes and infertility** – previous use of an IUD in nulliparous women is not associated with tubal factor infertility; however, untreated chlamydial infection is.
- **Partners will be aware of the presence of the IUD during sexual intercourse and it will cause pain** – the IUD threads rarely cause discomfort and soften with ongoing use. The IUD will not be dislodged by sexual intercourse. There is no reason why an IUD should negatively affect sexual pleasure or cause pain or discomfort during sex.
- **Women who are at risk of infective endocarditis cannot have an IUD** – the presence of risk factors for endocarditis such as valvular heart disease are not contraindications to IUD use and prophylactic antibiotics are not required for insertion or removal of IUDs.

EXAMPLE

A 28 year old with a 6 month history of irregular bleeding attends clinic requesting an IUD.

What questions do you ask? Would you insert an IUD?

1. History and nature of the bleeding.
2. Cervical screening history.
3. Past medical history.
4. STI risk assessment.
5. Examination of the cervix and STI screen, depending on the history.
6. Refer for assessment if bleeding continues and investigations are negative.
7. At present do not insert the IUD but offer an alternative until the bleeding is investigated.

References

British Association for Sexual Health and HIV (2019) *UK National Guideline for the Management of Pelvic Inflammatory Disease*. Clinical Effectiveness Group. [www.bashhguidelines.org/current-guidelines/systemic-presentation-and-complications/pid-2019/ – accessed May 2023]

British National Formulary, March 2023–September 2023.

FSRH (2022) *Service Standards for Resuscitation in Sexual and Reproductive Healthcare Services.*
[www.fsrh.org/documents/fsrh-service-standards-for-resuscitation – accessed May 2023]

FSRH (2023) *Clinical Guideline: intrauterine contraception*. Clinical Effectiveness Unit.
[www.fsrh.org/standards-and-guidance/fsrh-guidelines-and-statements/method-specific/intrauterine-contaception – accessed May 2023]

Heinemann, K. *et al*. (2015a) Risk of uterine perforation with levonorgestrel-releasing and copper intrauterine devices in the European Active Surveillance Study on Intrauterine Devices. *Contraception*, **91**: 274–279.

Heinemann, K. *et al*. (2015b) Comparative contraceptive effectiveness of levonorgestrel-releasing and copper intrauterine devices: the European Active Surveillance Study for Intrauterine Devices. *Contraception*, **91**: 280–283.

Office for National Statistics (2009) Opinions Survey Report No. 41 *Contraception and Sexual Health*, 2008/09.

UKMEC (2016) *UK Medical Eligibility Criteria for Contraceptive Use*
[www.fsrh.org/ukmec – accessed May 2023]

Chapter 10
Barrier methods

Barrier methods of contraception include male and female condoms, diaphragms and cervical caps. The male condom is used by just under 8% of couples globally and is the fourth most common birth control method worldwide. Caps and diaphragms are used by less than 1% of couples worldwide. In England, 14% of women report using the male condom as their main method of contraception, while less than 1% report using the female condom.

- Male condoms fit over an erect penis and female condoms are worn in the vagina – both act as a barrier to ejaculate, pre-ejaculate and cervicovaginal secretions.
- Female condoms consist of a loose sheath with an inner ring at the closed end; this is placed in the vagina. The second ring on the rim of the sheath covers the vulva (*Figure 10.1*).
- Both the cervical cap and diaphragm cover the cervix and spermicide should be applied to the device before insertion. They provide a physical barrier to sperm reaching the cervix.

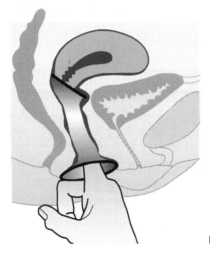

Figure 10.1 Positioning a female condom.

10.1 Potential users

10.1.1 Most appropriate users

- Male condoms can be used by almost everyone.
- Male and female condoms are not only a barrier method of contraception but also provide protection against STIs.
- Female condoms, diaphragms and cervical caps are most suitable for women who are comfortable with touching their genitals because they need to be inserted into the vagina.
- Barrier methods are ideal for couples spacing their family and in those where an unplanned pregnancy would be accepted.

10.1.2 Not suitable for the following users

- Couples who require a highly effective contraceptive. They may wish to use an additional method.
- Male condoms may not be suitable for men with erectile dysfunction. Their partner may prefer to use another contraceptive method.
- Those with a true latex allergy. However, they could try male or female condoms made from polyurethane.
- Diaphragms and caps may not be suitable for those with:
  - a history of toxic shock syndrome
  - an unusually shaped or positioned cervix because placement may be difficult
  - a sensitivity to spermicide
  - recurrent urinary tract infections
  - recurrent vaginal infections
  - HIV – due to the risk associated with the spermicide rather than the device itself; nonoxynol-9 may increase the risk of HIV transmission
  - a recent pregnancy or second trimester abortion; women are advised to wait 6 weeks post-delivery before caps and diaphragms are sized and fitted.

10.2 Available barrier methods

10.2.1 Male condoms

- Male condoms are made from latex, polyurethane, synthetic polyisoprene, or deproteinized latex.
- Some condoms are pre-lubricated.
- There are a variety of sizes, flavours and shapes available.
- Some condoms fit an individual better than others and so there is an element of trial and error for each individual in finding the best option.
- There is no evidence that condoms lubricated with spermicide (nonoxynol-9) provide additional contraceptive protection when compared with condoms lubricated with a non-spermicide. Nonoxynol-9 may also increase STI transmission as a result of its irritant effect.
- Male condoms reduce the risk of STI transmission when used for oral, anal and vaginal sex.

10.2.2 Female condoms

These are made of polyurethane, latex or nitrile, and are usually pre-lubricated with a non-spermicidal lubricant.

10.2.3 Diaphragms and caps

Table 10.1 shows the diaphragm and caps available in the UK, either directly from the manufacturers or via the internet for the women wishing to use the method. They must be used with a spermicide.

Table 10.1 Diaphragms and caps

	Presentation	Brand	Size	Cost
Diaphragm	Silicone – flexible rim	Caya	One size (fits women who require 65–80 mm diaphragm)	£49.85 for the device plus £16.88 for gel*
Cap	Silicone	Femcap	22, 26, and 30 mm	£15.29

* For personal purchase direct from manufacturer [accessed March 2023]
Other data from *BNF*, 2023.

- Diaphragms lie diagonally between the posterior fornix and pubic bone.
- Flat spring, coil spring and arcing spring diaphragms have been discontinued. While Milex wide-seal omniflex and arcing are still being produced, they are no longer listed in the *BNF* and are becoming increasingly more difficult to obtain.
- The flexible ring diaphragm is a single size which is suitable for approximately 80% of women. It is recommended that women are assessed prior to use to ensure the diaphragm fits correctly.

10.3 Efficacy

Table 10.2 shows the efficacy of each of the barrier methods.

Table 10.2 Percentage failure rate of each barrier method

Method	Percentage failure rate	
	Typical	Perfect
Female condom	21	5
Male condom	13	2
Caya	18	12
Femcap	14	8

- An unplanned pregnancy may occur with use of male and female condoms if:
  - they are fitted after genital touching has occurred
  - there are tears in the condom
  - a male condom slips off or penetration occurs outside the outer ring of the female condom
- The efficacy of diaphragm and cap can be reduced if:
  - it is damaged, for example, if a tear or hole is present
  - the incorrect size of device is used and therefore the cervix is not covered
  - it is used without a spermicide
  - inserted 2 or more hours before sexual intercourse for Caya (3 or more for other diaphragms)
  - it is removed too soon after sex, i.e. less than 6 hours
  - it is used for repeated episodes of sex without the application of additional spermicide.

10.4 Mechanism of action

- Barrier methods stop sperm and ovum meeting. They provide a barrier to the ejaculate and pre-ejaculate and work by preventing fertilization.

10.5 Pros and cons of barrier methods

10.5.1 Advantages

- Only need to be used when having sex.
- Provide protection for both partners against STIs (condoms).
- Are a non-hormonal method.
- Have no serious side-effects.
- Condoms, diaphragms and caps are available in a variety of sizes.
- Male condoms are easily available.
- Non-latex barriers are available.
- A female condom can be inserted up to 8 hours before sex.
- Female condoms are less likely to tear than the male condom.
- Diaphragms and caps can be inserted several hours before intercourse so that spontaneity can be maintained.
- The woman can control the use of contraception.
- Barrier methods are not compromised by concurrent drug therapy (for example, liver enzyme inducing drugs).
- Male condom use can increase the rate of human papillomavirus clearance and cervical intra-epithelial neoplasia regression.

10.5.2 Disadvantages

- Barrier methods require motivation to ensure use with each sexual episode.
- Barrier use may interrupt sex.
- Barrier methods are less effective than hormonal or intrauterine contraceptives.
- Latex sensitivity may occur (rare).
- Male condoms must be worn before there is any intimate contact.
- Male condoms may break or slip off during sex.
- Male condoms must be removed from the penis before it becomes flaccid.
- When using female condoms the penis must be inserted through the outer ring and not between the condom and vagina.
- Female condoms can slip out or be pushed into the vagina.
- The inner ring of the female condom may cause discomfort during sex.
- Female condoms can be noisy during sex.
- Women must be comfortable with self-examination in order to insert and remove female barrier methods.
- Diaphragms and caps cannot be used until 6 weeks post-partum or 6 weeks after a second trimester abortion.
- Diaphragms and caps do not reduce the risk of transmission of STIs.
- Women may find diaphragms and caps messy and dislike the idea of leaving them in place for 6 hours after sex.

10.6 Practical aspects

10.6.1 Male condoms

- Ask users to check the 'use by' date and safety markings (kite marks or CE mark) on the packet to ensure they meet appropriate recognized standards for strength and quality.
- The condom should be carefully removed from the packet to ensure it does not become damaged.
- A new condom should be used for each new episode of sexual intercourse.
- The closed end (teat) of the condom should be squeezed to expel any air.
- The condom is rolled down over an erect penis.
- It may be more comfortable for men with a foreskin to put the condom on after the foreskin is retracted. This enables the foreskin to move more freely during sex and it reduces the risk of the condom slipping off or tearing.
- After ejaculation and before the penis become flaccid the penis is withdrawn from the vagina with the bottom of the condom held in place to reduce slippage.
- The condom is then removed and disposed of in the bin rather than down a toilet.

Potential problems with male condoms

- Potential users should be advised that latex condoms (but not polyurethane condoms) may be damaged by oil-based lubricants, such as body oil or lotion, cooking oil, baby oil, suntan lotion or petroleum jelly.
- Oil-based preparations can damage latex condoms and make these methods less effective. These products include:
  - Canesten pessaries and cream
  - Cyclogest
  - Dalacin cream
  - E45 and similar preparations
  - Ecostatin
  - Fungilin
  - Gyno-Daktarin
  - Gyno-Pevaryl/Monistat
  - Nizoral
  - Witepsol-based products
- For anal intercourse the use of a water-based lubricant is recommended as it reduces the risk of breakage by 18%.

10.6.2 Female condoms

- Ask users to check the 'use by' date and safety marking on the packet.
- Carefully remove the condom from the packet to ensure it does not become damaged.
- The female condom can be inserted into the vagina any time up to 8 hours before sex.
- To insert the condom women are advised to find a position which is comfortable, such as lying down, squatting or with one leg elevated on a chair.

- Holding the closed end of the condom the inner ring is squeezed between thumb and finger.
- The labia are parted and the condom, along with the inner ring, is inserted into the vagina.
- The condom is then pushed up into the vagina so that the inner ring lies just above the pubic bone.
- The outer ring of the condom remains outside the vagina and lies up across the vulva.
- During sex the penis should be guided into the vagina through the centre of the outer ring of the condom.
- After sex the penis is withdrawn from the condom while the outer ring of the condom is held in place.
- The condom is removed by twisting the outer ring to ensure the semen remains within the condom, then pulling the condom out of the vagina and disposing of it in the bin.

10.6.3 Diaphragms

- Traditionally women wishing to use a diaphragm were examined and the correct size of diaphragm chosen; the size of the diaphragm equated to the approximate distance from the posterior fornix to the pelvic arch of the pubic bone. The largest size which felt comfortable, was ideal.
- Now women can purchase Caya (*Figure 10.2*) and self-fit without the need to see a healthcare professional.
- Caya is available in one size and fits 80% of women. It corresponds to traditional diaphragm sizes of 65, 70, 75 or 80 mm.
- Women can have the positioning of their diaphragm assessed at a sexual health service or general practitioner.
- The diaphragm should be positioned so that the rim fits comfortably into the posterior fornix, and the anterior rim should sit in the groove behind the pubic bone (*Figure 10.3*). Women are advised to self-assess the position of their Caya to ensure that their cervix is completely covered.

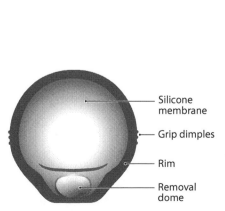

Silicone membrane

Grip dimples

Rim

Removal dome

Figure 10.2 Caya diaphragm.

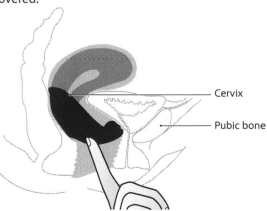

Cervix

Pubic bone

Figure 10.3 Correct position of inserted Caya diaphragm.

- It is recommended that women insert and remove the diaphragm on a few occasions prior to using it for sex, to ensure they are confident and comfortable with the method.
- Before sex the diaphragm should be checked to make sure there are no holes or tears.
- Before insertion, Caya is folded on the marked grip dimples. This creates dents or folds in the membrane of the diaphragm into which about 4 ml or one teaspoon of Caya Gel is applied (or two 2 cm strips of spermicide for other diaphragms). A small amount of the gel can be spread on the rim to aid insertion.
- Holding the diaphragm in one hand using the grip dimples, the diaphragm is inserted into the vagina with the woman in a comfortable position – be that standing, squatting or lying down. The diaphragm is gently pushed along the posterior vaginal wall until the cervix sits inside the diaphragm, with the edge of the removal dome sitting behind the pubic bone. Women are advised to use their finger to check the position of their device over the cervix prior to use.
- The diaphragm is removed by hooking a finger under the removal dome of the diaphragm. The device is then pulled downwards and removed from the vagina.
- If sex occurs either after the diaphragm has been in place for more than 2 hours (3 hours for other devices) or if sex is repeated, application of additional spermicide is required while the diaphragm remains in place.
- The diaphragm must be left in place for at least 6 hours after sex but no longer than 24 hours unless sex has occurred in the preceding 6 hours (30 hours for other devices).
- Once the diaphragm is removed it can be washed with warm water and mild soap. It is then rinsed, dried and stored in its container.
- Caya should be replaced two years after first use.

10.6.4 Caps

- FemCap is available in three different sizes: 22 mm, 26 mm and 30 mm.
- A pelvic examination is undertaken to estimate the size of the cervix and exclude any contraindications to use. As a general rule the 22 mm cap is used for nulliparous women, the 26 mm for women who have been pregnant but have not delivered vaginally (including C-section, abortion or miscarriage) and the 30 mm for women who have had a full-term vaginal delivery.
- It is recommended that women insert and remove the FemCap on a few occasions prior to using it for sex, to ensure they are confident and comfortable with the method.
- Before sex the FemCap should be checked for holes or tears.
- Apply approximately ¼ of a teaspoon of spermicide to the dome of the FemCap (this will face the cervix), then apply approximately ½ a teaspoon of spermicide to the groove between the brim and the dome (this area will face the vagina).
- The FemCap should be inserted with the woman in a comfortable position – be that standing, squatting or lying down. To insert the FemCap squeeze the sides together and insert it into the vagina with the bowl up and the long brim entering the vagina first. The FemCap is pushed into the vagina until the dome fits snugly over the cervix (*Figure 10.4*). It is then held in place by suction.

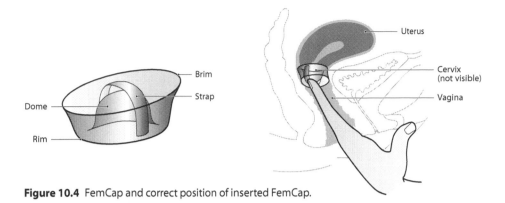

Figure 10.4 FemCap and correct position of inserted FemCap.

- The FemCap is designed with a longer brim which prevents it from being dislodged during sex. It is designed to rotate.
- To remove the FemCap locate the removal strap, rotate the device in a direction which is comfortable, and with relaxed muscles press on the dome to release the suction. This will enable women to hook the removal strap with their finger. The device is then withdrawn from the vagina.
- Once the FemCap is removed it can be washed with warm water and mild soap. It is then rinsed, dried and stored in its container.
- If sex occurs either after the FemCap has been in place for more than 3 hours or if sex is repeated, application of additional spermicide is required while the FemCap remains in place.
- The FemCap must be left in place for at least 6 hours after sex but no longer than 48 hours.
- A FemCap should be replaced 1–2 years after first use.
- A review is recommended following any pregnancy to re-assess the cervix and decide if a different size FemCap is needed.

Potential problems with diaphragms and caps

- The use of diaphragms and caps during menses is not recommended due to the potential risk of toxic shock syndrome.
- If vaginal dryness is experienced, water-based lubricants can be used with both Caya and FemCap.
- Following a vaginal infection women are advised to replace their device.
- Women who suffer from recurrent UTIs when using a diaphragm should be advised to empty their bladder before and after sex. Alternatively, change to using a cervical cap.
- In users complaining of vaginal soreness:
  - the size of diaphragm should be checked
  - investigate and treat any infection
  - consider a latex allergy
  - consider using Caya diaphragm and Caya diaphragm gel (non-spermicidal gel containing lactic acid).

- If a partner can feel the diaphragm the healthcare professional should:
  - check that the correct size is being used and that the cervix is covered
  - consider changing the type of diaphragm or to a cervical cap.

10.7 Myths and misconceptions

- **Discolouration of the diaphragm means it needs to be replaced** – this is incorrect; discolouration is normal but the functionality of the device is unaffected. Holes and tears, however, do affect the efficacy of the diaphragm and if either are found, the device should be replaced.
- **Both partners will be able to feel the diaphragm or cap during sex** – this is incorrect; if the correct size is used and the device is inserted correctly neither partner should be able to feel the diaphragm or cap. If the diaphragm or cap can be felt or is uncomfortable, a review is recommended, and if the problem continues an alternative cap or diaphragm or alternative method of contraception could be tried.
- **A condom will not roll all the way to the end of the penis and so all condoms are too small** – this is incorrect; the most likely explanation is that the condom is inside out and so it should be removed and a new one tried.
- **Using two condoms provides increased protection** – this is not only incorrect but actually increases the chances of method failure, as friction between the condoms raises the likelihood of them both tearing. In addition a male and female condom should not be used at the same time. Furthermore, lubricant should not be applied inside a condom (gel-charging) as this can result in the condom slipping off.
- **Condoms cause premature ejaculation** – this is incorrect; a male condom does not cause premature ejaculation. In fact, wearing a condom may reduce sensation and be helpful. Furthermore, some condoms contain a small amount of lidocaine gel to help prevent premature ejaculation.

EXAMPLE

A 26 year old women presents with genital irritation which she suspects is due to her partner's condom.

What would your management plan be?

1. Confirm whether the irritation may be due to condom use – consider differential diagnoses such as a dermatological condition, for example, eczema or dermatitis.
2. Determine the type of condom used; is it lubricated with a spermicide? Reactions to spermicides are more common than latex allergy.
3. Advise changing to polyurethane or deproteinized latex condoms or consider using a diaphragm or cap.
4. Most cases of latex allergy are mild with reactions occurring 24–48 hours following exposure and limited to the site of contact. Very rarely, symptoms become generalized. Repeated exposure may increase the risk of a reaction occurring.
5. Occasionally further investigation is warranted with skin testing for the presence of immunoglobulin E antibodies against latex.

References

British National Formulary, March 2023–September 2023.

FSRH (2012, updated 2015) *Barrier Methods for Contraception and STI Prevention*. Clinical Effectiveness Unit.
[www.fsrh.org/standards-and-guidance/documents/
ceuguidancebarriermethodscontraceptionsdi – accessed May 2023]

Chapter 11
Fertility awareness

Fertility awareness is the generic term for what is colloquially known as the 'rhythm method' or 'using the safe period'. Using signs of the fertile phase of the menstrual cycle, pregnancies can be planned and also potentially avoided without the use of additional hormones or devices.

In the UK about 2% of couples use fertility awareness as their method of contraception, but worldwide many more use these methods to space their families. Natural family planning is effective if couples abstain from penetrative sex or use barrier methods during the fertile phase of the menstrual cycle.

'Withdrawal' (removing the penis from the vagina before ejaculation) is used by 4% of British couples as their method of contraception. This is seen by many to be a 'natural' method and will be discussed in more detail at the end of the chapter.

11.1 Potential users

11.1.1 Most appropriate users

- Couples wanting to use a natural contraceptive method with no hormones or interruption of sex.
- Women who have a regular menstrual cycle.
- Couples willing to consistently keep a diary, recognize the signs of the fertile phase and understand the importance of abstaining from sex or using barrier methods during this phase.
- Couples need to be highly motivated.
- These methods are ideal for couples who want to space their children and where an unplanned pregnancy would be accepted.

11.1.2 Not suitable for the following users

- Those requesting or requiring a highly effective method of contraception.
- Women who are taking teratogenic drugs.
- Women for whom pregnancy would put them at high risk of serious morbidity or mortality.
- Women with irregular menstrual cycles.
- Women who are post-partum and not breastfeeding.
- Women who are peri-menopausal.
- Women who have recently discontinued a hormonal contraceptive method. They should only rely on data once periods have returned and they have had a minimum of three regular cycles.
- Fertility awareness is not suitable for women who find it difficult to follow the instructions for recognizing the fertile phase or could not abstain or use barrier methods during this time.
- Withdrawal is not suitable for men:
  - who could not recognize the pre-ejaculatory phase
  - who may not comply on all occasions.

11.2 Available fertility awareness methods

These are summarized in *Table 11.1*.

Table 11.1 Fertility awareness methods in common use

Method	How it is used	What is required	How much does it cost?
Temperature	The basal body temperature is measured each morning before getting up	A sensitive digital thermometer	About £10
Calendar	This is recorded over a 12 month period to calculate the longest and shortest cycles	Calendar downloaded from www.fertilityuk.org/	No cost
Cervical mucus	Changes during the month are noted	Correct technique	No cost
Two day method	Avoid having sex if cervical secretions are noted on the day of observation and the day before	Correct technique	No cost
Symptothermal method (using a combination of methods)	Different fertility indicators are used; normally the menstrual calendar, body temperature and cervical mucus	Correct technique and documentation (fertility awareness calendar) plus thermometer	About £10
Lactational amenorrhoea method (LAM)	When a woman is fully breast-feeding within 6 months of the baby's birth	Correct technique	No cost
Devices for detecting fertile phase	Devices detect the fertile phase by measuring urinary estriol-3-glucuronide and LH	Monitors and testing sticks	£15–£93
Fertility apps such as Natural Cycles and watches such as AVA	Apps and watches track the menstrual cycle and body temperature	Correct technique and documentation	Natural Cycles costs £59.99 a year and AVA £249

Costs checked March 2023 amazon.co.uk and providers.

11.3 Mechanism of action

Sperm survive up to 7 days in the cervical mucus during the fertile phase and an ovum will be receptive to fertilization for 24 hours. Therefore the fertile phase is thought to last up to 9 days (see *Figure 11.1*). Any method that can detect this fertile phase so that couples can either abstain or use a barrier method during this time may help prevent a pregnancy.

The withdrawal method requires a man to remove his penis from the vagina before he ejaculates.

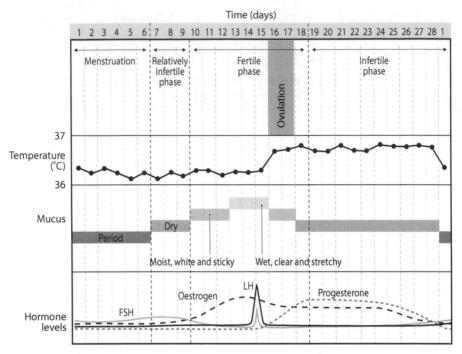

Figure 11.1 Signs used for fertility awareness methods when using the symptothermal method (a combination of the calendar method, basal body temperature and cervical secretions).

11.4 Efficacy

- The fertile window can vary from month to month. Therefore couples are required to avoid sex or use barrier methods for 8–9 days each month, even if they are using a number of fertile phase indicators.
- The failure rate using one indicator can be as high at 23%, but as low as 0.4% when using the symptothermal method (a combination of the calendar method, basal body temperature and cervical secretions).
- Devices such as Persona, watches such as AVA and apps such as Natural Cycles detect the fertile phase, giving a typical failure rate of about 8%.
- Withdrawal has a failure rate of 4% with perfect use and 20% in typical use because the pre-ejaculate has been shown to contain motile sperm in many men.

11.5 Pros and cons of fertility awareness

11.5.1 Advantages

- Can be used to plan pregnancy as well as prevent conception.
- No known physical side-effects.
- Non-intercourse related method.
- No mechanical devices or hormones used.

- Acceptable to all cultures and religions.
- Once learnt by the user no further follow-up is necessary.

11.5.2 Disadvantages

- Has a relatively high failure rate in practice when using only one fertility awareness indicator.
- Requires commitment from both partners.
- Illness may affect body temperature readings.
- Successful use depends on education.
- Requires careful observation and record keeping, which may take time to learn.
- Users must have high motivation, as there are often long periods of abstinence from intercourse or use of barrier methods.
- Does not protect against sexually transmitted infections.
- Does not offer the advantages of hormonal methods in reducing menstrual loss and dysmenorrhoea or endometrial/ovarian cancer.

11.6 Using the different methods

11.6.1 Temperature

- Once ovulation has occurred, progesterone is produced by the corpus luteum; this causes the basal body temperature to rise.
- Using a sensitive digital thermometer the woman takes her temperature daily before getting up and following at least 3 hours of rest.
- The post-ovulatory infertile phase can be detected by measuring a rise of 0.2°C on three consecutive days when compared to the previous six days.
- No additional method of contraception is needed once the post-ovulatory infertile phase has been identified until the start of menstruation.
- Using this method alone couples will need to avoid sex or use barrier methods for about 16 days each month (days 3 to 19 in a typical 28 day cycle): this is during the whole of the pre-ovulatory phase.

11.6.2 Calendar method

- Normally 12 months of menstrual cycle data should be documented to accurately predict the fertile phase each month.
- The fertile phase when using the calendar method only normally lasts up to 16 days and abstinence or use of an additional method is required during this time (days 8 to 19 on a 28 day cycle).
- The shortest and longest cycle should be used to calculate the fertile period.
- The first fertile day is determined by subtracting 20 days from the shortest cycle.
- The last fertile day is established by subtracting 10 days from the longest cycle.
- The fertile phase should be constantly adjusted using data from the last 12 months.

- The simplified calendar method is a simpler method for those women with regular cycles between 26 and 32 days (see *Figure 11.2*).

Simplified calendar method
Women should have cycles between 26 and 32 days (no irregular cycles) The first fertile day will always be day 8 The last fertile day will be day 19 Abstinence or barrier methods are required between day 8 and day 19 each month

Figure 11.2 Simplified calendar method.

11.6.3 Changes in cervical secretions and cervix

- During the ovulatory phase of the cycle women produce more oestradiol from the developing ovarian follicle which results in cervical secretions becoming abundant, stretchy and similar to raw egg white mid-cycle.
- Women need to record when they first notice any secretion and this is the start of the fertile phase. At this time the couple need to abstain or use a barrier method.
- Once the secretions have reached their peak day, where they will be similar to raw egg white, the secretions then become thicker and less abundant under the influence of progesterone. When this change has been present for a full 3 days the fertile phase ends and no additional method is required.
- Changes to the cervix may also indicate the fertile phase but should only be used in conjunction with other indicators.
- When the cervix feels high, soft and open (low, soft and open if the uterus is retroverted), sex should be avoided or barrier methods used.
- No additional methods are needed when the cervix is low, firm and closed (high, firm and closed for women with a retroverted uterus) for 3 consecutive days.
- Use of barrier methods and spermicides may interfere with the use of cervical secretions as a fertile phase indicator. Other indicators, therefore, should also be used.

11.6.4 Two day method

- This is a modification of the cervical secretion method and is simple to learn.
- Secretions should be assessed in the late afternoon or evening.
- Abstinence or use of barriers is required when secretions are seen on the day of observation or the day before.
- Once there have been two consecutive dry days no additional methods are required.

11.6.5 Devices, watches and apps for detecting the fertile phase

- There are devices that detect the fertile phase by measuring urinary estriol-3-glucuronide and luteinizing hormone (LH).

- When increased levels of these hormones are measured, abstinence or additional barrier methods should be used.
- Watches such as AVA record a number of physiological parameters, including skin temperature, pulse rate and sleep patterns. These are analysed on a back-end server and results sent to the user's smartphone.
- Apps such as Natural Cycles use an algorithm which calculates the fertile window from basal body temperature and menstrual calendar data. Up to 60% of days in the first cycle may require abstinence or barrier methods, decreasing to 30% after several cycles.

11.6.6 Lactational amenorrhoea method (LAM)

Breastfeeding is a natural way to space children. Suckling suppresses LH and FSH, which results in amenorrhoea and stimulation of prolactin leading to lactation. LAM is very effective, offering 98% protection against pregnancy when the following conditions exist:
- A woman is fully or almost fully breastfeeding (feeding with no substitutes and at regular periods on demand, day and night)
- There are no long intervals between feeds, e.g. no more than 4 hours during the day and 6 hours during the night
- The baby is less than 6 months old
- Menstruation has not returned.

11.7 Withdrawal method

'Withdrawal' is the oldest method of birth control; it is still one of the most popular natural contraceptive methods worldwide. It can be practised by any couple at any time.

11.7.1 Advantages of withdrawal

- It is free of charge.
- It requires no prescription.
- It does not cause nausea or weight gain.
- It is acceptable to many users.

11.7.2 Disadvantages of withdrawal

- It has a high failure rate.
- Sex is often thought to be incomplete.
- It may be unsatisfying for either or both parties.
- Partial ejaculation of semen can occur resulting in failure of the method.
- It does not protect against STI/HIV transmission.

11.8 Myths and misconceptions

- **Fertility awareness is complicated and difficult to teach** – no it is not. Women with regular cycles who are motivated to use these methods can find all the necessary information on the internet. Instruction guides are available along with downloadable charts and a digital thermometer can be bought. Barrier methods are then used until a woman has enough data to accurately predict her fertile phase. See www.fertilityuk.org for further details.
- **Using fertility awareness as a contraceptive method results in a high risk of pregnancy** – this is not correct. Couples who consistently use several fertility indicators, such as with the symptothermal method, have a failure rate of just 0.4%.
- **Couples using withdrawal should be advised to use condoms to reduce their chance of an unplanned pregnancy** – there is no evidence to support this advice. Many couples are happy using withdrawal and often feel pressurized to change their method. The typical failure rates of withdrawal and condoms are similar, therefore couples should choose the method that most fits their needs.

EXAMPLE

A 28 year old woman is having problems working out her fertile phase using the calendar method. She has recorded her periods over the last 12 months with the shortest cycle from the first day of one period to the first day of the next being 24 days. Her longest cycle is 32 days.

What do you advise?

1. She can use the Standard days method to work out the first day of her fertile phase by taking 20 from her shortest cycle (24 days). Therefore her first fertile day is day 4 of each cycle.
2. Her last fertile day is calculated by subtracting 10 from her longest cycle (32 days). Therefore her last fertile day is day 22.
3. She would then have to abstain from sex or use an additional contraceptive method for 19 days each month.
4. To help shorten the fertile phase she may therefore use a second or even third indicator, such as using her basal body temperature or cervical secretions.

References

FSRH (2015) *Fertility Awareness Methods*. Clinical Effectiveness Unit. [www.fsrh.org/documents/ceuguidancefertilityawarenessmethods/ – accessed June 2016]

Office for National Statistics (2009) Opinions Survey Report No. 41 *Contraception and Sexual Health*, 2008/09.

Urrutia, R.P. and Polis, C. (2019) Fertility awareness based methods for pregnancy prevention. *BMJ*, **366**: 76–79.

Chapter 12
Male and female sterilization

Worldwide, sterilization is the most common method of contraception; female sterilization is used by 19% of women aged 15–49 who are married or in a relationship, and male sterilization is used by 2% of men worldwide. There are two methods of sterilization available in the UK: vasectomy for men and laparoscopic sterilization for women. In England, there were just over 12 000 vasectomies and just under 14 000 laparoscopic sterilizations performed in 2017/18.

12.1 Potential users

Sterilization is a permanent method of contraception suitable for all those who do not wish to have children or have completed their family.

12.1.1 Most appropriate users

Male and female sterilization can be used by the majority of men and women. It is most suitable for those who have completed their families and have had no surgery to the abdomen or testicles.

12.1.2 Not suitable for the following users

There are few conditions which would completely restrict an individual's eligibility to undergo sterilization; however, a delay may be recommended until the patient is medically fit for surgery or an experienced surgeon is available.

The procedure is normally conducted in a surgical day unit, but there may be certain circumstances which require extra preparation, precautions and counselling. For example:
- obesity (BMI >35) makes the procedure more difficult, and there is increased risk of wound infection and complications at time of surgery
- uterine fibroids may make it more difficult to localize the Fallopian tubes
- large varicocele or hydrocele may make localizing the vas deferens more difficult.

For certain medical conditions, or following a related procedure, it may be more prudent to delay the procedure until the condition is evaluated, treated and/or changes or resolves. For example:
- post-abortion – it is advisable to delay sterilization until 6 weeks post-abortion, with the provision of alternative contraception in the interim
- current infection – it is advisable to allow time for effective treatment of the infection, be that pelvic inflammatory disease, epididymitis or sexually transmitted infection, or gastrointestinal or respiratory infection.

For other conditions it may be advisable that the procedure is undertaken in a setting with an experienced surgeon and staff, the equipment needed to provide general anaesthesia or undertake additional/alternative procedures, as well as access to back-up medical support. For example:
- for a woman with a fixed uterus due to previous surgery or infection – the risk of laparotomy is increased and complications are more likely.

Alternative temporary methods of contraception should be provided, if referral is required or there is any other reason for a delay.

12.2 Available methods of sterilization

These are summarized in *Table 12.1.*

Table 12.1 Summary of methods of sterilization

Method	Typical anaesthetic requirement	Time from procedure until current or additional contraception can be stopped
Vasectomy	Local	Once semen sample is negative for sperm – typically tested 12 weeks post-vasectomy
Laparoscopic tubal occlusion	General or regional – usually as a day case	Immediately effective so long as there are no viable sperm in the genital tract – contraception should be continued for at least a week

12.3 Mechanism of action

- Sterilization interrupts or occludes the passage of sperm or ovum.

12.4 Pros and cons of sterilization

12.4.1 Advantages

- Non-hormonal method.
- Removes the need for future/ongoing contraception.
- No hormonal side-effects.
- Rarely has a long-term effect on health.
- No effect on libido or sexual function.

12.4.2 Disadvantages

- A surgical procedure is required.
- Uncommonly, the vas deferens or Fallopian tube(s) may re-join, returning an individual to fertility, possibly leading to an unplanned pregnancy.
- Sterilization cannot be easily reversed and reversal is not available on the NHS.
- Sterilization does not protect against STIs.
- The production of a semen sample will be required about 12 weeks after the procedure, and ongoing contraception will be needed until tests confirm that the semen sample is sperm-free.
- Each method is associated with potential complications.
- There may be regret associated with the permanence of the procedure, particularly if circumstances change.

12.5 Counselling and consent

Discussion prior to sterilization is ideally undertaken with both partners present and encompasses the following:

- Ensuring that both partners do not want children, or if they already have children that their family is complete. Enquire about number of children, if they have family with their current partner, and if there are any circumstances in which they may wish to have a future pregnancy.
- Identify reasons for the sterilization to ensure that the method is appropriate and that there is no coercion on the part of either partner.
- Ask about past medical and surgical history; for example, a history of endometriosis, abdominal or testicular surgery which may affect the feasibility of the procedure. In addition, ask about any current conditions, such as anticoagulant use, which may require an alternative procedure or additional precautions during surgery.
- Current contraception – advice can be given regarding likely change in periods once this method is stopped.
- Menstrual history – which may suggest more applicable alternative methods of contraception; for example, a history of heavy menstrual bleeding for which a levonorgestrel IUS would be an effective method of managing symptoms and providing long-term contraception.
- Failure rate.
- Discussion of other highly effective methods such as LARCs.
- Irreversibility.
- Time until the procedure is effective and the minimum length of time that current reliable contraception should be continued. There is no need to stop CHC prior to surgery.
- Details of the available procedures including the associated risks, benefits, recovery, complications and myths and the type of anaesthetic required. Provide written information to support the details given in the consultation; these can be accessed from www.rcog.org.uk or www.nhs.uk.
- Inform both partners that, compared to female sterilization by laparotomy or laparoscopy, vasectomy:
  - is more effective
  - is safer
  - is quicker to perform
  - is associated with less morbidity
  - requires only a local anaesthetic.
- These methods provide no protection against STIs.
- Male or female genital examination is advised to exclude potential problems such as a hydrocele, non-palpable vas deferens, gynaecological pathology, or evidence of previous surgery.

12.6 Regret

Evidence indicates that men and women are more likely to regret sterilization if they were under 30, had had no children, were not in a relationship, had relationship problems, or were sterilized immediately post-partum or post-abortion. In light of this, young and single people often receive additional counselling and may need to be reviewed by two specialists (rather than the typical one) before the procedure is undertaken.

Emotional problems including psychosexual dysfunction are more likely post-procedure if an individual is not absolutely certain about their decision at the time of the procedure.

12.7 Practical aspects

12.7.1 Vasectomy

This method of sterilization aims to prevent sperm entering the ejaculate through interruption of the vas deferens.

Efficacy
- Late failure due to re-joining of the ends of the tubes after initial negative semen analysis and resulting return to fertility occurs in approximately 1:2000 male sterilizations.
- Early failure, wherein post-operative semen analysis shows persistent motile sperm, occurs in approximately 1:250 male sterilizations.
- Compared to laparoscopic female sterilization, vasectomy is 30 times less likely to fail and 20 times less likely to be associated with post-operative complications.

Procedure

There are a variety of techniques for vasectomy, two of which are outlined below. Irrespective of the method chosen, the procedure typically takes 10–15 minutes to complete.

Conventional vasectomy:
- The scrotal skin is anaesthetized and two small incisions approximately 1 cm long are made.
- The incision provides access to the vas deferens which is cut and a small section removed. The ends of the vas deferens are ligated with sutures or cauterized.
- The incision is then closed, often with absorbable sutures such as Vicryl Rapide.

Minimally invasive vasectomy (MIV) (incorporating no-scalpel vasectomy (NSV) techniques):
- The vas deferens is located by palpation. Following infiltration with local anaesthetic, the vas deferens is held in place by a small clamp.
- The skin of the scrotum is punctured on one side and forceps are used to open the incision site. A loop of vas deferens is then drawn through the incision. The vas

deferens is interrupted and a section (1–3 cm long) is removed. Routine histological analysis of the removed section is not recommended.

- The upper and lower ends of the divided vas deferens are ligated or cauterized. Fascial interposition can be undertaken as an adjunctive procedure.
- The second vas deferens can be accessed, divided and ligated or cauterized through the original puncture site.
- With this approach the opening in the scrotum is very small and may not require sutures to close.

The MIV techniques (as shown in *Figure 12.1*) are thought to be less painful and less likely to cause post-operative complications than a conventional vasectomy. Furthermore, cauterization is associated with a lower failure rate than ligation. The failure rate can be reduced by about 50% with fascial interposition (rate based on semen analysis).

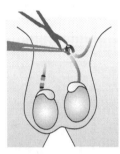

Figure 12.1 MIV vasectomy.

Post-procedure advice
- Men are advised to take a day or two off work if they have a sedentary job and up to a week off for those who have a manual job.
- Abstinence from sexual intercourse is recommended for 2–7 days.
- Firm scrotal support in the form of well-fitting underwear should be worn day and night for the first few days to reduce the risk of haematoma development.
- NSAIDs can be taken for post-operative pain unless there are personal contraindications.
- A post-vasectomy semen analysis should take place a minimum of 12 weeks after surgery and after a minimum of 20 ejaculations. Assessment of a single sample is acceptable to confirm vasectomy success if all recommendations and laboratory methodology are met and no sperm are observed.
- Advice to contact a healthcare provider if there is persistent bleeding, pain, possible infection or rapidly enlarging one-sided scrotal haematoma is routinely given.

Risks and complications
- Mild testicular discomfort, swelling and/or bruising are common in the first few days following a vasectomy and can generally be managed by simple analgesics.
- Haematospermia (blood in semen) is common in the first few ejaculates after a vasectomy.

- Scrotal haematoma (minor bleeding 1:400, major bleeding 1:1000).
- Infection (1:100).
- Epididymitis (1:100).
- Sperm granuloma (1:500) – typically a small hard mass or lump which may be symptomatic or asymptomatic and is due to sperm leaking from the vas deferens into the surrounding tissue. Most sperm granulomas resolve by themselves. They are commonly treated with NSAIDs but if particularly large or painful, may require surgical removal.
- Chronic pain or post-vasectomy pain syndrome (1:1000) can develop immediately following vasectomy or months to a year later. The pain is long-standing but not necessarily constant. It may occur occasionally or more frequently and can vary from a dull ache to a sharp pain. NSAIDs and treatment to alleviate neuropathic pain are common first-line treatment options. When this fails, further surgery involving reversal of vasectomy may be required, although pain may persist in a few cases.
- Failure to identify or locate one of the vas deferens – unilateral vasectomy can be undertaken followed by semen analysis at 12 weeks post-procedure. Referral for renal ultrasound to exclude ipsilateral renal agenesis is recommended.
- Where apparent bilateral absence of the vas deferens is encountered:
  ○ men should be referred for further investigation
  ○ if a double or duplicate vas deferens is found or suspected, arrange Doppler ultrasound to determine if it is a 'true' double vas deferens or an ectopic ureter. A renal and bladder ultrasound should also be arranged.
- There is currently no evidence of a causal relationship between vasectomy and prostate cancer and no increased risk of testicular cancer.
- Failure of the procedure has occurred if motile sperm are still seen 7 months post-surgery. In a small minority of men non-motile sperm are found in a specimen 7 months after vasectomy. Special clearance can be given to stop additional contraceptive methods when less than 100 000 non-motile sperm/ml are observed in two fresh semen samples.
- Late failure due to vas recanalization occurs in 0.03–1.2% of previously effective vasectomies.

12.7.2 Laparoscopic sterilization (tubal occlusion)

This method of sterilization involves preventing an ovum reaching the uterus through occlusion or interruption of the Fallopian tubes.

It can be undertaken at any time providing the woman attending has abstained from sexual intercourse since her last menstrual period or is correctly using an effective method of contraception. If there is concern regarding a potential pregnancy the procedure should be delayed until the follicular phase of the next menstrual cycle.

Efficacy

- The lifetime failure rate for laparoscopic sterilization is up to 1 in 200.
- The 10 year failure rate for sterilization using Filshie clips appears to be lower at 2–3 per 1000.

- Patients should be aware that if the procedure fails there is an increased risk of ectopic pregnancy.

Procedure

- Pre-operatively a pregnancy test is undertaken along with recording of last menstrual period and current method of contraception. Risk of a potential pregnancy is likely to result in postponement of the procedure.
- A standard laparoscopic approach is taken, with insufflation of the abdomen and then insertion of a port sub-umbilically. Once the laparoscope is passed through the port site the abdominal wall can be visualized and a second port can be introduced under direct vision in the suprapubic region.
- The Fallopian tubes are then identified and clips are applied across the narrowest portion of the tube, 1–2 cm from the cornu, to occlude the Fallopian tubes. Alternatives to clips include rings, ligation, salpingectomy or diathermy.

Mini-laparotomy

A mini-laparotomy is an alternative approach.

- A small transverse incision just above the pubic symphysis (typically 4 cm above) is made.
- The Fallopian tubes are identified and a small portion removed (salpingectomy) or the tubes are occluded with clips or rings.
- There is less chance of reversal with tubal diathermy or salpingectomy than with other techniques.

A mini-laparotomy may be recommended for women who:
- Have had recent abdominal or pelvic surgery.
- Are obese.
- Have a history of pelvic inflammatory disease.
- Immediately post-partum or if the procedure is undertaken at the time of caesarean section. Both Filshie clips and modified Pomeroy technique are effective.
- As an alternative if a laparoscopic approach fails.

Post-procedure advice

- Women should be informed of the method of sterilization which has been undertaken.
- The majority of women return home on the day of the procedure.
- Women are advised to take 5–7 days off work depending on their occupation.
- If any intra-operative complications occur during the procedure both the patient and GP should be informed, along with information about the method used to undertake the sterilization.
- If abdominal pain increases, fever develops or an individual feels increasingly unwell they are advised to seek urgent medical help because these symptoms may suggest an infection or perforation to bowel, bladder or blood vessels.
- Contraception – women using CHC, the POP or non-hormonal contraception should be advised to continue their contraceptive method for at least 7 days after laparoscopic sterilization. The IMP can be removed at the time of the procedure or

any time following the procedure. If an IUC is *in situ* it should remain until at least 1 week post-procedure.

Potential complications

- Women who are obese, have significant pathology, have had previous surgery or have a pre-existing medical condition should be advised that the quoted risks for significant or frequent complications may be increased.
- Failure to gain entry into the abdomen.
- Injury to bowel, bladder and or blood vessels (2–3 per 1000); this risk is increased in obese women, those with adhesions or endometriosis, those who have previously undergone abdominal or pelvic surgery or have pelvic inflammatory disease.
- Risk of death with laparoscopy is 1 in 12000 procedures.
- Uterine perforation (1:1000).
- The risk of laparotomy following laparoscopic tubal occlusion is up to 3 in 1000.
- Infection.
- Haemorrhage.
- Bruising.
- Abdominal and shoulder pain is common and normally caused by the creation of a pneumoperitoneum during surgery. This gradually settles during the week following the procedure.
- Moderate to severe abdominal pain is reported in up to 63% of women post-operatively, with 27% of women experiencing milder pain, and 50% experience mild pain at 3 months post-procedure.
- There is no evidence that sterilization results in heavier or more painful periods; however, women have often used hormonal methods of contraception prior to their sterilization which lightens menstrual loss and decreases dysmenorrhoea.
- Failure of procedure. If the procedure fails, any resulting pregnancy may be ectopic.
- If reversal of sterilization for pregnancy is requested, patients can pay for a Fallopian tube re-anastomosis, as this procedure is not funded by the NHS; this procedure is associated with high tubal patency rates, but this may still not result in a pregnancy.

12.7.3 Hysteroscopic sterilization

Essure is a form of female sterilization which involves the hysteroscopic insertion of flexible micro-inserts into the proximal section of the Fallopian tubes and is undertaken without general anaesthesia. In 2017 Essure was discontinued from the UK for commercial rather than safety reasons; therefore hysteroscopic sterilization is no longer available. Women who have already undergone this procedure do not need to take any action unless they have pain or ongoing problems.

12.8 Myths and misconceptions

- **Vasectomy causes cancer** – there is no evidence of a causal relationship between vasectomy and prostate or testicular cancer.
- **Vasectomy causes weight gain, hair loss or reduced strength** – vasectomy has no effect on male hormone levels; men look and feel the same as prior to the procedure.
- **Vasectomy results in a loss of sexual function and sex drive** - vasectomy does not affect the sexual drive, nor does it affect a man's ability to achieve an erection, have sex, or ejaculate. In fact, now that the risk of pregnancy has been removed sexual pleasure may actually increase.
- **Vasectomy alters the amount and appearance of the ejaculate** – this is not true because most of the ejaculate is made up of secretions from the seminal vesicles, prostate gland and Cowper's glands; this does not change post-vasectomy – only the sperm are absent.
- **Vasectomy reversal is always effective** – vasectomy reversal requires complex surgery and although high patency rates are achieved, a return to fertility may not occur. The longer the duration from vasectomy to reversal, the lower the patency and pregnancy rates.
- **Female sterilization causes cancer** – sterilization does not increase the risk of cancer; indeed, several studies have reported a reduced risk of ovarian cancer after tubal occlusion. Very little research has been done to investigate the relationship between breast cancer and female sterilization, but so far there is no evidence of such a link.
- **Female sterilization stops ovulation and affects hormones** – sterilization acts to block the Fallopian tubes to prevent the ovum entering the uterus. It does not prevent ovulation. In addition, female hormones are not affected and so there is neither a loss of femininity nor any change in sexual functioning.
- **Female sterilization causes periods to become more painful, heavier or more irregular** – as sterilization has no effect on hormonal function there is no effect on an individual's menstrual cycle. Women often use hormonal contraceptives prior to sterilization which generally lightens periods and helps period pain. Women notice changes in their periods due to the absence of hormonal contraception, not the presence of the sterilization.
- **Female sterilization causes weight gain and loss of sex drive** – there is no evidence that sterilization affects weight, appetite or physical appearance; however, weight gain is more common in older women and this group is more likely to undergo sterilization. Sterilization has no effect on sexual desire or function – in fact women may find sexual pleasure increases once they do not have to worry about pregnancy risk.

EXAMPLE

A 39 year old woman who has 2 children attends requesting sterilization because she is looking for a long-term method of contraception. She has a past medical history of endometriosis which has been investigated with a laparoscopy.

What questions you would ask and what are the management options?

1. Ideally you would see the woman with her partner.
2. Take a complete medical and surgical history, along with current contraception and current gynaecological symptoms. Determine the paternity of her children and ensure her family is complete.
3. Identify reasons for requesting the sterilization.
4. Discuss alternatives to sterilization such as LARC.
5. Discuss advantages, disadvantages and potential complications of the methods.
6. If sterilization is chosen as the method of contraception, vasectomy would be the safest option in this case. If laparoscopic sterilization is the selected option, then surgery should be undertaken by an experienced surgeon as there is an increased risk of laparotomy and complications are more likely.

References

DeBono, M.A. (2016) *Female Sterilisation* (Consent Advice No. 3) RCOG. [www.rcog.org.uk/en/guidelines-research-services/guidelines/consent-advice-3 – accessed May 2023]

FSRH (2014) *Male and Female Sterilisation*. Clinical Effectiveness Unit. [www.fsrh.org/standards-and-guidance/documents/cec-ceu-guidance-sterilisation-cpd-sep-2014 – accessed May 2023]

Hancock, P., Woodward, B.J., Muneer, A. *et al.* (2016) Laboratory guidelines for postvasectomy semen analysis: Association of Biomedical Andrologists, the British Andrology Society and the British Association of Urological Surgeons. *Journal of Clinical Pathology*, **69**: 655–660.

NHS Digital (2018) *Sexual and Reproductive Health Services, England – 2017/18*. [https://digital.nhs.uk/data-and-information/publications/statistical/sexual-and-reproductive-health-services/2017-18#summary – accessed May 2023]

Sokal, D., Irsula, B., Hays, M. *et al.* (2004) Vasectomy by ligation and excision, with or without fascial interposition: a randomized controlled trial. *BMC Med*, **2**: 6. [https://bmcmedicine.biomedcentral.com/articles/10.1186/1741-7015-2-6 – accessed May 2023]

Chapter 13
Emergency contraception

Emergency contraception (EC) is taken after sex has occurred, to prevent an unintended pregnancy. It is also known as post-coital contraception or the 'morning after pill'. EC is used by 7% of women each year in the UK. Because no method of contraception is perfect, EC is an important back-up for all. Accessing EC is often felt to be difficult due to the stigma women perceive to be associated with its use.

There are three forms of EC currently available in the UK:
- oral progestogen-only EC – levonorgestrel
- oral selective progesterone receptor modulator – ulipristal acetate (UPA)
- copper IUD.

In the UK oral EC is available from community pharmacies (provision is free in Scotland and Wales and in many pharmacies in England under 'Patient Group Direction' issuing; however, in some pharmacies individuals may be charged between £10.00 and £30.00), GP surgeries, sexual and reproductive health clinics and genitourinary medicine clinics. Oral EC may also be available from young people's services, school nurses, accident and emergency departments, NHS walk-in centres (England only), NHS minor injuries units and online pharmacies.

In addition, IUDs are available free of charge from sexual and reproductive health clinics, young people's services (where registered nurses are employed) and GP surgeries.

EC may be needed because contraception was not used, or because of a contraceptive failure such as forgotten progestogen-only or combined contraceptive pills, expulsion of an intrauterine contraceptive or because of failure of a barrier method (see *Tables 13.2* and *13.3* later in this chapter for possible indications for EC). EC is not an abortifacient and, with the exception of the copper IUD, does not provide ongoing contraception.

Previously, a combined (oestrogen and progestogen) oral preparation known as the Yupze method was used; however, this is less effective than progestogen-only EC and is no longer available in the UK. Mifepristone may be used as an EC; however, it is not licensed in the UK.

13.1 Potential users

13.1.1 Most appropriate users

- All women with no contraindications should be offered an IUD because it is the most effective method of EC.
- There are no medical contraindications to levonorgestrel EC.

13.1.2 Not suitable for the following users

The copper IUD is not suitable for those:
- more than 2 days but less than 4 weeks post-partum (although fitting may be considered by specialist services depending on circumstances)

- with persistently elevated β-hCG levels following gestational trophoblastic or malignant disease
- with uterine cavity distortion – an attempt may be undertaken after careful counselling
- with current pelvic inflammatory disease
- with a history of copper allergy
- with known long QT syndrome
- with known symptomatic *Chlamydia trachomatis* infection or current *Neisseria gonorrhoeae* infection.

Liver enzyme inducing drugs (see *Table 3.1*) increase the metabolism of both LNG and UPA, which may reduce their effectiveness. Therefore an IUD is the method of choice for those using these medications. However, if an IUD is contraindicated or declined, a double dose (3 mg) of LNG can be prescribed (off licence) along with an explanation

Table 13.1 EC available in the UK

Method	Cost	Recommended dose	Licensed indication
Copper-bearing IUD	Prices vary from £8.00 to £15.20	1 device which can be retained until pregnancy excluded, e.g. onset of period or at least 3 weeks after unprotected sex, or up until the licensed duration of the IUD	Within 5 days (120 hours) of first episode of unprotected sex or within 5 days of the earliest estimated date of ovulation, whichever is later
Levonorgestrel (progestogen)	*Emerres* – Drug tariff £5.20 (£3.65 NHS indicative price) *Levonelle 1500* – Drug tariff £5.20 (£5.20 NHS indicative price) *Levonorgestrel* – Drug tariff £5.20 (£3.74– £5.20 depending on manufacturer NHS indicative price) *Melkine* – Drug tariff £5.20 (£5.20 NHS indicative price) *Upostelle* – Drug tariff £5.20 (£3.75 NHS indicative price)1 tablet	1.5 mg single oral dose	Within 72 hours of unprotected sex or contraception failure or, off licence, up to 96 hours after unprotected sex; however, efficacy decreases with time
Ulipristal acetate (UPA) (progestogen receptor modulator)	*ellaOne 30 mg tablets* – Drug tariff £14.05 (£14.05 NHS indicative price) *Ulipristal generic* – Drug tariff £14.05 (£13.35– £17.50 NHS indicative price)	30 mg single oral dose	Within 120 hours of unprotected sex or contraception failure

Data from *BNF*, 2023.

that the effectiveness of this approach is not known. A double dose of UPA is not recommended.

UPA is not recommended for women who are:
- hypersensitive to UPA
- severe asthmatics treated by oral glucocorticoids
- galactose intolerant, lactase deficient or have glucose–galactose malabsorption
- breastfeeding (feeding not recommended for 7 days after UPA use – the milk should be expressed and discarded).

Oral EC preparations contain lactose.

13.2 Available emergency contraception in the UK

Doses, indications and the cost of EC products are provided in *Table 13.1*.

13.3 Mechanism of action

13.3.1 Copper IUD

- The main mode of action when used as EC is inhibition of fertilization. If fertilization has already occurred, the IUD has an anti-implantation effect.
- It is effective immediately as an ongoing method of contraception.

13.3.2 Levonorgestrel

- The mechanism of action is not completely understood but is thought to be primarily by the delay or prevention of ovulation. Ovulation is delayed for 5 days by which time any sperm in the reproductive tract will be non-viable.
- When taken prior to the onset of the luteinizing hormone (LH) surge, ovulation is delayed or inhibited (see *Figure 13.1*).
- If fertilization has occurred, LNG has no effect on pregnancy prevention. It is not known to adversely affect pregnancy outcome.

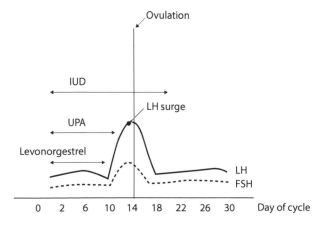

Figure 13.1 Efficacy of EC in relation to ovulation. The lines on the graph indicate the times during which a method is most likely to be effective. If the LH surge has not yet started all three methods may be effective in preventing pregnancy. Once the LH surge has started only UPA and the IUD are beneficial. Following the LH peak an IUD is efficacious.

- Women may ovulate later in the cycle. It is important women are aware of this, to enable them to make decisions about contraception options.
- LNG is licensed for use up to 72 hours after unprotected sex, but it may be taken up to 96 hours after unprotected sex (off licence).
- Resume or start contraception with additional barrier method cover as outlined in *Table 13.4*.

13.3.3 Ulipristal acetate (UPA)

- UPA is a selective progesterone receptor modulator with antagonistic and partial agonistic effects. It binds to progesterone receptors in target tissues: the uterus, ovaries and hypothalamus.
- Its main mode of action is to delay ovulation for at least 5 days. If the LH surge has started but not peaked, ovulation can be inhibited, with up to a 5 day delay in follicular rupture. The majority of women will ovulate later in their current cycle. It is important women are aware of this, to enable them to make decisions about their contraceptive options.
- Administration at the time of or after the peak of the LH surge has no effect in delaying follicular rupture.
- Women should wait 120 hours after using UPA before starting or recommencing hormonal contraception, as current evidence suggests concurrent use may reduce the efficacy of the UPA. During this time and until effective contraceptive cover from their chosen method of contraception has been achieved (see *Table 13.3*) individuals should either abstain or use barrier methods.

13.4 Efficacy of emergency contraception

Studies suggest that the pregnancy rate with the different types of EC varies as follows:
- following LNG use the estimated pregnancy rate is 0.6–2.6% if UPSI occurred within the previous 72 hours
- following UPA use the estimated pregnancy rate is 1–2%. There is no decline in efficacy over time up to 120 hours after UPSI; however, the effectiveness of UPA in delaying ovulation may be reduced if a woman takes progestogen in the 5 days after taking UPA, and the efficacy of UPA could theoretically be reduced if progestogen has been taken in the week prior to taking UPA
- following the use of an IUD as EC very few women become pregnant (<0.1%); one large study of nearly 2000 women reported no pregnancies in the first month after EC IUD fitting.

Ideally, therefore, an IUD should be offered first-line to all women who have no contraindications. Furthermore, an IUD is the only method of EC that is effective post-ovulation.

The efficacy of oral EC may be reduced in women with a greater weight. For women with a BMI >26 kg/m² or a weight of >70 kg LNG is less effective. For women with a BMI >30 kg/m² or a weight of >80 kg, UPA is also less effective. Data is limited but current advice is that if an IUD is declined, UPA can be offered and if this is not suitable then

3 mg of LNG (double dose, both tablets taken at the same time) is recommended for women with a BMI >26 kg/m².

The metabolism of both UPA and LNG is increased by liver enzyme inducing drugs. This may reduce their effectiveness of oral EC, therefore an IUD is the method of choice. A double dose (3 mg) of LNG can be taken by women using enzyme inducers, although its effectiveness is not proven. A double dose of UPA is not recommended.

13.5 Provision of emergency contraception

When assessing the need for EC it is important to consider:
- LMP date
- the need for a pregnancy test
- usual cycle length and estimated date of ovulation. Ovulation occurs about 14 days prior to onset of menstruation. The earliest likely ovulation date is the start date of the LMP plus 14 days less than the number of days in the shortest cycle. 5 days are then added to this date to determine the latest date an IUD can be fitted. In order to determine this estimated date, LMP must be accurately known and a woman's cycle must be regular. *Figure 13.2* provides a different approach to estimating date of ovulation.
- the timing of **all** episodes of unprotected sex in the current cycle (see *Table 13.2*)

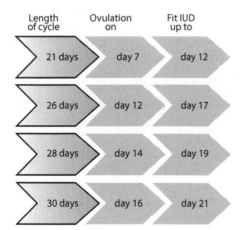

Length of cycle	Ovulation on	Fit IUD up to
21 days	day 7	day 12
26 days	day 12	day 17
28 days	day 14	day 19
30 days	day 16	day 21

Figure 13.2 How to calculate the period of time when an EC IUD can be fitted.

Table 13.2 Indications for emergency contraception for women not currently using a method of contraception

Situation	Indication
Women not using contraception	women who do not wish to conceive should be offered EC after UPSI that has taken place on any day of a natural menstrual cycle
After pregnancy	women who do not wish to conceive should be offered EC for: • UPSI from day 21 following childbirth (unless the criteria for lactational amenorrhoea are met). IUC can be offered from day 28 • UPSI from day 5 after an abortion, miscarriage, ectopic pregnancy or uterine evacuation for gestational trophoblastic disease

- details of potential contraceptive failures, for example, how many missed pills and when in the packet (see *Table 13.3*)
- previous EC use in the cycle

Table 13.3 Indications for emergency contraception in current users of contraception

Method of contraception	Possible contraceptive failure	Indications for EC
Combined hormonal or progestogen-only pill or implant	Failure to use additional contraceptive precautions whilst using liver enzyme inducing medication or in the 28 days following their use	If unprotected sex has occurred or barrier method fails Use IUD or double dose LNG (3mg)
Combined oral contraceptive	Two or more missed pills	EC is indicated if the pills were missed in week one of a packet and unprotected sex occurred during that 1st week or during the hormone-free week EC is indicated if the HFI is extended; an IUD can be fitted up to 13 days after the last active pill (providing all other pills had been taken correctly) Theoretically the effectiveness of UPA-EC could be reduced if CHC has been used in the 7 days prior to EC, therefore consider LNG-EC or an IUD
Combined contraceptive ring or patch	Extension of patch or ring-free interval by more than 48 hours If patch or ring is detached or removed for more than 48 hours	EC is indicated if sex occurred in the patch- or ring-free interval; an IUD can be fitted up to 13 days after the start of the HFI EC should be considered if the patch or ring was detached or removed in week 1 and unprotected sex occurred in the patch- or ring-free week Theoretically the effectiveness of UPA-EC could be reduced if CHC has been used in the 7 days prior to EC, therefore consider LNG-EC or an IUD
Progestogen-only pill	Late or missed pills, i.e. more than 27 hours since last traditional POP or more than 36 hours since last desogestrel-containing POP	EC is indicated if there has been unprotected sex or a barrier failure since the missed pill and before efficacy is re-established, i.e. in the 48 hours after starting the POP; an IUD can be fitted up to 5 days after the first episode of unprotected sex or oral EC can be offered Theoretically the effectiveness of UPA-EC could be reduced if POP has been used in the 7 days prior to EC use, therefore consider LNG-EC or an IUD
Progestogen-only injectable	Late injection more than 14 weeks since last injection of DMPA	EC is indicated if all unprotected sex occurred in the last 5 days – an IUD may be fitted or oral EC used Theoretically the effectiveness of UPA-EC could be reduced by residual circulating progestogen, therefore consider LNG-EC or an IUD, depending on the history
Intrauterine methods	Removal without immediate replacement, partial or complete expulsion	If sex occurred in the 5 days before removal or expulsion, offer oral EC Depending on an individual's history it may be appropriate to fit an IUD

- past medical history to determine medical eligibility
- medications used, including herbal medicines which may affect efficacy of oral EC
- the need for ongoing contraception, which should be discussed with all women attending for EC
- sexual history to determine symptoms and STI testing requirements (see *Chapter 14*).

All methods of EC which are appropriate to the clinical circumstances should be offered and discussed, including their effectiveness, to enable women to select their preferred method.

- An IUD is the most effective option and therefore is generally first-line.
- To maximize the likelihood that oral EC is taken before ovulation, it should be taken as soon as possible after UPSI.
- Take a pragmatic approach to providing oral EC. UPA-EC can be considered the first-line oral EC for women:
  - who had UPSI 96–120 hours ago (even if there has been UPSI within the last 96 hours)
  - who have had UPSI within the last 5 days if the UPSI is likely to have taken place during the 5 days prior to the estimated day of ovulation
  - for whom it is not possible to establish a likely date of ovulation.
- If an individual presents requiring EC between 72 and 120 hours after sex, but UPA is contraindicated and an IUD is declined, LNG may be used but its efficacy will be reduced. There is evidence suggesting that LNG-EC has no effect after 96 hours.
- If a woman presents more than 5 days after the most recent UPSI it is unlikely that oral EC will be effective. If an IUD is declined, offer immediate quick start of contraception with a follow-up pregnancy test in 3 weeks.
- Another important consideration is the need for ongoing contraception and how this may affect choice of oral EC. A clinician is advised to consider the relative risks and benefits of providing an immediate quick start of a contraceptive method along with LNG rather than UPA and a delayed start of a method of contraception.
- If a woman presents requesting EC or is identified as requiring EC more than once in the cycle it is important to provide it. There is a significant risk of pregnancy when oral EC has been provided earlier in the cycle leading to postponed ovulation. If all episodes of UPSI were within 5 days of an estimated date of ovulation, an IUD can be used. If an oral method is requested, LNG and UPA can be used more than once in a cycle. However, if a woman has already taken UPA-EC, LNG-EC should not be taken in the following 5 days, and if a woman has already taken LNG-EC, UPA-EC could theoretically be less effective if taken in the following 7 days. In these instances a repeat of the original oral EC or an IUD is advised.
- Oral EC can be provided even if other episodes of UPSI have occurred earlier in the cycle (>5 days prior to presenting). Neither method of oral EC is known to affect an ongoing pregnancy or lead to fetal abnormality. If there was UPSI more than 21 days prior to their attendance, a high sensitivity pregnancy test should be undertaken prior to providing EC.

If a woman selects an IUD as her method of EC but it is not immediately available, oral EC should be given as an interim measure in case the IUD cannot be fitted or the woman fails to attend the appointment. To facilitate this process clear referral pathways are advised.

13.6 Provision of ongoing contraception

- The EC consultation provides an opportunity to discuss future contraception.
- Women may select an IUD for EC and ongoing contraception.
- Women may prefer to wait until pregnancy can be excluded before starting a hormonal method. It is important women are aware that there is a risk of pregnancy if further episodes of UPSI occur during their cycle.
- Quick-starting an ongoing method of contraception (see *Chapter 2*) after EC can be considered for all women based on their medical eligibility and preference. *Tables 13.4* and *13.5* illustrate the duration of additional contraception following use of LNG-EC and UPA-EC. Note that following UPA use, the chosen method of contraception should not be commenced until 5 days (at least 120 hours) after EC.
- It is recommended that the progestogen-only injectable is quick-started only if all other methods are declined.

Table 13.4 Duration of additional contraceptive or abstinence required following use of LNG-EC

Method of contraception started or recommended	Duration of additional contraception or abstinence or abstinence following use of LNG-EC
CHC including patch and vaginal ring	7 days
COC containing oestradiol valerate and dienogest	9 days
Progestogen-only implant	7 days
Progestogen-only injectable	7 days
Progestogen-only pill	2 days

Table 13.5 Duration of additional contraceptive or abstinence required following use of UPA-EC

Method of contraception started or recommended	Delay required after UPA use before contraception can be started or recommended	Duration of additional contraception or abstinence following use of UPA-EC
CHC including patch and vaginal ring	UPA given on Day 0 Advise women not to commence contraception until Day 5 after UPA use (120 hours after UPA)	7 days
COC containing oestradiol valerate and dienogest		9 days
Progestogen-only implant		7 days
Progestogen-only injectable		7 days
Progestogen-only pill		2 days

> ### EXAMPLE
>
> **A 30 year old woman attends to discuss contraception because she wishes to start 'the pill'. Her LMP was 12 days earlier; it was a normal period. She typically has a 28 day cycle, has no medical conditions or contraindications and is not currently using any medication. She had a condom failure 2 days ago (day 10).**
>
> *What should you discuss?*
>
> 1. Check if any other episodes of unprotected sex have occurred during this cycle.
> 2. Any use of EC earlier in this cycle?
> 3. Sexual history to determine risk and offer STI testing as appropriate.
> 4. Discuss all EC options available: IUD, LNG and UPA.
> 5. Carefully discuss the efficacy of each method, explaining that the IUD is the most effective method of EC.
> 6. If she opts for an oral method, LNG would be an acceptable option.
> 7. If she wishes to quick-start an oral method of contraception following LNG-EC, a POP could be commenced with additional contraception for 2 days or, if a CHC is preferred, 7 days of additional contraception would be required.
> 8. Follow-up for pregnancy test in 3 weeks.

- The IUS should not be quick-started but a bridging method used until pregnancy can be excluded.

13.7 Aftercare

- For women who commence a contraceptive method following EC, a pregnancy test 21 days after last (most recent) UPSI is recommended.
- A pregnancy test is recommended if the next menstrual period is delayed by more than 7 days, is lighter than usual or is associated with abdominal pain that is not typical of the woman's usual dysmenorrhoea.
- Consider repeating offer of STI screening.
- If pregnancy occurs following oral EC, women can be reassured that evidence suggests there is no harmful effect on pregnancy outcomes and no increase in the risk of congenital abnormality. (For advice on pregnancy with IUD *in utero* see *Chapter 9*.)
- Once pregnancy has been excluded, an IUD may be removed once ongoing contraception has been established or in line with standard IUD removal (see *Chapter 9*).

13.8 Managing side-effects

- Nausea occurs in fewer than 20% of women following oral EC and vomiting in less than 1%. If vomiting occurs within 3 hours of taking UPA or LNG a further dose of EC is needed or an IUD could be fitted.
- The time of menses may be affected by EC. Most women bleed within 7 days of their expected period date. Menses may be earlier or later than expected; the timing of menses is affected by when within the cycle the EC is taken. Women should be advised that fewer than 1 in 5 women have a period that is delayed for 7 days or more with UPA. If menses is delayed by more than 7 days following the use of EC, a pregnancy test is recommended.
- Pain associated with insertion of an IUD may occur and this can generally be alleviated with simple analgesia and advice to return if pain fails to resolve or becomes severe.
- Other side-effects associated with oral EC include headache, dizziness, diarrhoea and breast tenderness, which all resolve quickly after use.

13.9 Myths and misconceptions

- **There is only one type of emergency contraception and it can only be used the morning after unprotected sex** – there are three methods of EC currently available in the UK and, potentially, they may all be suitable depending on the timing of unprotected sex. UPA and the IUD can be offered up to 5 days after unprotected sex.
- **Emergency contraception causes an abortion** – this is not correct; EC works by delaying ovulation or preventing fertilization or implantation and so its action occurs before implantation occurs, which is legally when pregnancy begins. Religious and cultural beliefs may be different and should be respected.
- **Emergency contraception causes infertility** – EC has a very short-term effect and there is no effect on future fertility.
- **Emergency contraception can only be used a small number of times in a woman's life** – there is not a maximum number of times EC can be used. EC can be used whenever it is needed. Frequent use of oral EC is not recommended, however, because it is not as effective as regular contraception but repeated use poses no health risks and has no effect on future fertility.
- **Emergency contraception should not be provided as an advanced supply** – this is not the case; research suggests that women who have EC in advance are more likely to use it and use it sooner after the episode of sex than those without an advanced supply. While routine advanced supply would not be cost-effective, the provision of an advanced supply can be decided on a case-by-case basis for women who may be at risk; for example, those women using barrier methods or the withdrawal method.
- **If pregnancy occurs after emergency contraception use it needs to be managed differently to any other pregnancy** – for those who had an IUD inserted, the site of pregnancy should be determined by ultrasound scan and

removal of the IUD before 12 weeks of pregnancy is recommended. An IUD left *in situ* during pregnancy is associated with miscarriage, preterm delivery, septic abortion and chorioamnionitis. Removal of the IUD improves outcome.

EXAMPLE

A 19 year old woman attends requesting emergency contraception. She had unprotected sex the night before. Discussion reveals her LMP was 17 days earlier and she has a 28 day cycle. She also had unprotected sex on days 15, 14 and 13.

What should you do?

1. Determine medical history to assess medical eligibility.
2. Sexual history to determine risk and offer STI testing as appropriate.
3. As all sex occurred within 5 days of estimated date of ovulation (estimated date of ovulation is day 14 in in a 28 day cycle therefore an IUD could be fitted up to day 19), an IUD would be the most appropriate method of EC and may also be used for ongoing contraception.
4. Organize IUD fit if acceptable. Provide UPA if there are no contraindications and an IUD fitting cannot be undertaken immediately.
5. In an asymptomatic woman insertion of an IUD can be carried out without the need for prophylactic antibiotics, providing she is easily contactable and will re-attend if an infection is identified.
6. Prophylactic antibiotics for chlamydia (and gonorrhoea depending on local prevalence) can be considered in those at high risk of an STI.
7. Follow-up in approximately 3 weeks after next menses.

References

British National Formulary, March 2023–September 2023.

FSRH (2017, amended 2020) *Emergency Contraception*. Clinical Effectiveness Unit. [www.fsrh.org/standards-and-guidance/documents/ceu-clinical-guidance-emergency-contraception-march-2017 – accessed May 2023]

Chapter 14

STIs, safe sex and sexual assault

- Sexually transmitted infections (STIs) are infections passed from one person to another during sex or close sexual contact.
- The recognition of, and screening for, STIs are important components of sexual and reproductive health, irrespective of the setting in which a consultation takes place.
- There are no contraindications to the offer of testing for infections. In fact, if we offer testing as part of 'contraception' consultations, we increase the scope and acceptability of testing.

14.1 Potential users

Table 14.1 outlines the situations in which clinicians may wish to consider undertaking STI testing.

Table 14.1 When and to whom to offer STI testing

Situation	Description
On request from patient	• As part of sexual health many individuals now attend for a regular check-up based on their own perceived risk
Known at-risk individuals	• Under 25 years of age • New partner within the last 12 months • More than one partner in the previous 12 months • Intravenous drug user • From high-risk area for HIV or syphilis (e.g. sub-Saharan Africa, Russia and parts of South East Asia and the Caribbean) • Those who have paid for sex or who have been paid for sex • Those who have had a blood transfusion in the UK pre-1992 or surgery/transfusion abroad • Those who have high-risk partner, i.e. partner who has an STI, who has multiple sexual partners, who is bisexual, who uses intravenous drugs, or from high HIV or syphilis-prevalent country • Those who have a clinical indicator disease for HIV as outlined in the UK national guidelines for HIV testing, such as cervical intra-epithelia neoplasia grade 2 or above, oral candidiasis, pyrexia of unknown origin (see www.bhiva.org/HIV-testing-guidelines.aspx for further details)
Symptomatic patients	• With increase or change in vaginal discharge • With dysuria • With intermenstrual or post-coital bleeding • With pelvic or abdominal pain • With dyspareunia
Pre-procedure	• Before abortion • Before insertion of intrauterine contraception, endometrial sample, hysteroscopy in known at-risk groups
Screening programme	• Chlamydia screening programme for all sexually active women and men under the age of 25 years

14.2 Sexual history taking

A sexual history is important in the assessment of risk and in determining which infections to test for and from which sites. Sexual health issues may present as a hidden agenda in a consultation. Individuals may be reluctant to discuss their health concerns due to fears of stigma.

Components of a sexual history include:
- Symptoms review – change in vaginal discharge, dysuria, skin changes, abdominal or pelvic pain, intermenstrual or post-coital bleeding.
- Previous sexual partners – all partners in the last 3–6 months, time of last episode of sex, gender of partner(s), condom use, type of sex (anal, oral or vaginal).
- Previous STIs – diagnosis, treatment, compliance with treatment and treatment of partner. Is there a risk of re-infection or failure of treatment?
- Last menstrual period, cycle length, intermenstrual bleeding, post-coital bleeding, contraceptive use and cervical sample history.
- Blood-borne virus risk assessment, including history of blood transfusion (pre-1992), surgery, injection or blood transfusions outside the UK, intravenous drug use by self or partner, any other recreational drug usage, partner(s) from overseas, partner(s) who have sex with men, being paid or paying for sex, known blood-borne virus infection in partner.
- A means of providing the results of investigations, e.g. text, letter.
- Assessment for vulnerability, risk of exploitation or child protection concerns.

There are a variety of testing kits and several laboratory platforms available for infection testing.
- They differ with regard to transportation and refrigeration and so a discussion with local laboratory services is recommended.
- The gold standard tests and, where applicable, alternative tests for the most common infections are outlined in *Table 14.2* along with incubation periods and/or window periods, first-line treatment and recommended follow-up.
- While there is currently insufficient evidence to recommend routine screening for *Mycoplasma genitalium*, testing is recommended in the following circumstances: individuals diagnosed with non-gonococcal urethritis and pelvic inflammatory disease. Testing should also be considered for individuals with signs or symptoms of mucopurulent cervicitis (particularly post-coital bleeding), epididymo-orchitis or sexually acquired proctitis.
- Testing should not be delayed until the end of a window period. Instead individuals should be tested at time of presentation and advised of the need for repeat testing if last sexual partner was within the window period.

Table 14.2 Testing, window/incubation periods, treatment and follow-up for common STIs

Infection	Test	Window or incubation period since last UPSI	Treatment	Repeat testing
Chlamydia trachomatis	NAAT* – site determined by history	2 weeks	Doxycycline 100 mg orally twice daily for 7 days OR Azithromycin 1 g orally followed by 500 mg once a day for 2 days If pregnant or breast-feeding: • erythromycin 500 mg four times a day for 7 days OR • erythromycin 500 mg twice a day for 14 days OR • amoxicillin 500 mg three times a day for 7 days OR • azithromycin 1 g orally then 500 mg once a day for 2 days	Not routinely needed unless: • the woman receiving treatment is pregnant (due to reduced efficacy of treatment) • compliance issues are suspected Residual non-viable DNA may be detected by NAAT for 3–5 weeks after treatment
Neisseria gonorrhoeae	NAAT* – following positive diagnosis a culture specimen should be taken to enable identification of antibiotic sensitivity	2 weeks as infection cannot be ruled out in individuals who test within two weeks of sexual contact with an infected partner	Ceftriaxone 1 g single dose IM injection OR Spectinomycin 2 g single dose IM injection OR If antimicrobial susceptibility test results from all sites of infection are available prior to treatment and the isolate is sensitive to ciprofloxacin, then this should be used for treatment in preference to ceftriaxone. Ciprofloxacin 500 mg PO single dose OR Cefixime 400 mg orally as a single dose plus azithromycin 2 g orally, if IM injection is contraindicated or refused	A repeat NAAT swab is recommended 2 weeks after treatment if diagnosis is made by NAAT as a 'test of cure'

Infection	Test	Window or incubation period since last UPSI	Treatment	Repeat testing
Trichomonas vaginalis	NAAT* (or culture broth if NAAT not available); or wet mount microscopy if available; may be identified as part of cervical screening (smears) Point of care test – OSOM rapid test	Unknown; however, *in vitro* studies suggest 4–28 days Any partners within the 4 weeks prior to presentation	Metronidazole 400 mg orally twice a day for 7 days OR Metronidazole 2 g orally as a single dose (avoid single high dose in breastfeeding)	Not required unless the individual remains symptomatic after treatment
HIV	Clotted blood for both HIV antibodies and p24 antigen (a 4th generation HIV test): p24 antigen is a protein which makes up most of the viral core; concentrations of p24 are high in the first few weeks of infection; antibodies to p24 are produced following seroconversion and so p24 is generally undetectable after seroconversion after initial infection antibodies to HIV antigens begin to appear in the blood; screening test looks for antibodies to HIV surface proteins	4 weeks (8 weeks in high risk exposure; 8–12 weeks following an assault, the latter if PEP has been taken)	Anti-retroviral therapy depending on CD4 count and patient request	Monitoring and follow-up will depend on local and national guidelines
Syphilis	Clotted blood for serological testing to look for treponemal antibodies (including syphilis); a screening test or full syphilis serology may be requested: all individuals with	Incubation period 9–90 days; end of window period is 12 weeks after exposure	For early syphilis (primary, secondary or early latent) benzathine penicillin G 2.4 million units IM as a single dose OR doxycycline 100 mg orally twice daily for 14 days	Follow-up at 3, 6 and 12 months, then 6-monthly if indicated, until Rapid Plasma Reagin (RPR) test or the Venereal Disease Research Laboratory (VDRL) test are

(continued)

Infection	Test	Window or incubation period since last UPSI	Treatment	Repeat testing
Syphilis (cont'd)	previous infection with syphilis should always have a full syphilis screen (not always available in general practice). Syphilis PCR testing or dark ground microscopy on a swab taken from a chancre if identified on examination		For late syphilis: • benzathine penicillin 2.4 million units IM weekly for 3 weeks (three doses) OR • doxycycline 100 mg orally twice daily for 28 days	negative or serofast (levels or VDRL or RPR remain static); these are non-specific quantitative tests which correlate with disease activity
Genital warts (human papillomavirus)	Visual inspection or biopsy if any doubt about diagnosis	Variable but generally 3 weeks to 8 months	No treatment or • Excision • Electrosurgery • Cryotherapy • Podophyllotoxin topically twice a day for 3 days, followed by 4 days with no treatment for 4–5 cycles. • Imiquimod 5% – 3 times weekly for up to 16 weeks	Review at end of treatment or if change of treatment is required or if relapse occurs
Genital herpes (herpes simplex virus)	Visual inspection, NAAT* for confirmation and typing (use of serology for antibodies to herpes simplex virus is limited)	2–14 days, however, testing is only undertaken if symptomatic	• Saline baths • Analgesia • Topical anaesthetic (5% lidocaine ointment) • Aciclovir 400 mg orally 3 times a day for 5 days OR valaciclovir 500 mg orally twice daily (only indicated if presentation is within 5 days of start of episode), while new lesions are still forming	Not indicated

Infection	Test	Window or incubation period since last UPSI	Treatment	Repeat testing
Mycoplasma genitalium	NAAT*; positive specimens should be tested for macrolide resistance-mediating mutation	There is no data available on incubation period or likely window period; however, tests available are sensitive and likely to detect early infection. Testing of current partner is recommended	Doxycycline 100 mg twice a day for seven days followed by azithromycin 1 g orally as a single dose then 500 mg orally once daily for two days OR moxifloxacin 400 mg orally once daily for 14 days if organism is known to be macrolide-resistant or the woman has PID. Many individuals will be treated first time with doxycycline, for uncomplicated infection; a repeat course may not be needed once the *Mycoplasma genitalium* positive result is known. Azithromycin is ideally given immediately after doxycycline but can be given up to 2 weeks after doxycycline. If administration is later than 2 weeks after doxycycline the course of doxycycline should be repeated prior to azithromycin.	Repeat NAAT 6 weeks after completion of treatment as a 'test of cure'

*NAAT – nucleic acid amplification test

14.3 Partner notification

- An important public health component of STI testing is partner notification. Its aim is to reduce or stop the onward transmission of infection through the identification, testing and, if appropriate, treatment of others known to be at risk as a result of sexual contact with the index case (i.e. the individual who was initially diagnosed).
- The process of partner notification involves identifying a look-back interval during which the infection of contacts may have occurred, identifying contacts who may have been at risk of infection and agreeing who will inform the contacts, the index case or a healthcare provider, for example, in primary care or via a GUM clinic anonymously. Finally, follow-up of the outcomes of partner notification is recommended.

- The clinic or practice undertaking the initial testing and/or treatment does not necessarily need to complete the partner notification. However, discussion of the process involved and the importance of partner notification is recommended. A referral can be made to a local sexual health service which can facilitate the process of partner notification.
- There are many means through which partner notification may occur, including telephone call, text message, email, letter, contact slip and social media. The aim is to inform the contact of the need to attend a service for testing and, potentially, treatment. For example, "Please phone the health advisers at xxx hospital about an important matter concerning your health" or "This email is to inform you that you have been in contact with someone who has xxxx. This is a treatable condition and often people with this infection feel well and have no symptoms. It is very important that you are tested and treated if needed. Therefore please attend xxxx."
- Face-to-face or telephone consultations can be undertaken to provide support and advice to contacts about the possibility of infection and the provision of treatment if appropriate.

14.4 Sexual health advice

Safe sex is the means of taking responsibility for oneself by taking steps to reduce the risk of STIs and unplanned pregnancy. Sexual history taking can help identify those undertaking risky sexual behaviour who may benefit from a brief behaviour change intervention. Brief interventions have been shown to reduce STI incidence and increase condom usage.

Safe sex advice includes verbal and written information on:
- Condom efficacy and limitations (see *Chapter 10*).
- Condom types and sizes – ensure the condom is the correct size, particularly with regard to penis circumference, and is not too tight.
- Determinants of condom effectiveness.
- Use condoms for all episodes of sex including oral sex with advice that, while oral sex is lower risk than vaginal or anal sex, it is not risk free. If condoms are not used for every episode of sex, some use is safer than no use.
- STI testing is recommended before having sex with someone new and advising new partners to undergo testing even if they have no symptoms.
- Reducing the number of partners to reduce infection risk. This risk reduction, in terms of prevalence of infection, may be greater than that associated with increased condom use.
- Risk of transmission in penetrative sex including fingering, using sex toys and fisting relates to the degree of trauma experienced by an individual.
- Avoid brushing teeth or flossing before oral sex.
- Avoid oral sex if cuts, sores or cold sores (oral herpes) are present on the mouth of the individual giving oral sex or if that individual has a sore throat. While oral sex is lower risk than vaginal or anal sex it is not risk-free.

- In addition, a condom demonstration and discussion regarding condom problems can be beneficial. Issues to discuss include:
  - removing air from tip of the condom
  - pulling back foreskin before putting on the condom to reduce the risk of condom slipping off or tearing
  - use of additional lubricant may double the risk of condom slippage
  - thicker condoms are no less likely to break or slip during anal sex than standard condoms.
- In 2022 there was an increased number of Mpox cases (previously known as monkeypox). It can be passed from person to person through close physical contact and most cases have been in men who are gay, bisexual or have sex with other men (MSM). Incubation period is between 5 and 21 days, with symptoms including pyrexia, headache, muscle/joint pains, lymphadenopathy, fatigue and a blistering rash starting 1–5 days after initial symptoms, and it can be confused with chickenpox. Symptoms tend to be mild and usually clear up in a few weeks without treatment.
- Those concerned that they might have Mpox should contact their local sexual health clinic and are advised to stay at home, avoiding close contact with other people until they see a HCP.
- Vaccination is available and is being offered to healthcare workers caring for patients with confirmed or suspected Mpox, MSM, and men who have multiple partners, participate in group sex or attend sex-on-premises venues (staff at these venues are also eligible). It is also available to people who have been in close contact with someone who has Mpox – ideally, they should have 1 dose within 4 days of contact, but it can be given up to 14 days after contact. Healthcare workers will be offered 2 doses of the vaccine, as will MSM, with the 2nd dose given 2 to 3 months after the 1st dose.

14.4.1 HIV pre-exposure prophylaxis (PrEP)

- PrEP is an HIV prevention strategy and is indicated for those at greater risk of HIV acquisition. HIV-negative individuals take tenofovir and emtricitabine before they potentially encounter HIV. Evidence shows that this approach reduces HIV acquisition.
- Currently PrEP is available in Scotland through sexual health clinics, in Wales as part of the PrEPARED trial from a select list of sexual health or genitourinary medicine (GUM) clinics, in England as part of the PrEP IMPACT trial and in Northern Ireland as part of a pilot via a centralized service. In addition, PrEP can be purchased; see www.iwantprepnow.co.uk/buy-prep-now/
- For those resident in England and Northern Ireland who are not able to access clinical trials and cannot afford to purchase PrEP, the Terrence Higgins Trust has set up the Mags Portman PrEP Access Fund (MPPAF).
- Current recommendations are that PrEP is offered to the following HIV-negative individuals:

- ○ those who have condomless sex with an HIV-positive partner(s), unless the partner has been on ART for at least 6 months and their plasma viral load is <200 copies/ml
  - ○ MSM who have condomless sex
  - ○ trans women who have anal sex.
- While in the UK PrEP is not recommended for **all** women, national guidelines advocate that PrEP should be offered on a case-by-case basis, taking into account a person's circumstances determined as a result of history taking and risk assessment. Some groups of women at potentially increased risk of HIV include those whose partners are from high risk countries or population groups. In addition women who experience coercive power dynamics within their relationships, and who have little control over their condom use, might also be at enhanced HIV risk.
- Furthermore, PrEP should be considered on a case-by-case basis in trans women and trans men wherein current factors increase the risk of HIV acquisition.
- While on-demand dosing regimens are available for MSM, daily dosing is recommended for those having vaginal sex because all of the studies of on-demand dosing have involved only MSM. Tenofovir takes much longer to reach required level in vaginal as opposed to rectal tissue, meaning on-demand dosing is likely to be less effective.

14.5 Sexual assault

A compassionate and pragmatic approach is required when an individual presents following a sexual assault. An individual may attend immediately after the assault or after some considerable time, or at any point in between. The needs of the individual may be affected by the duration of time since the event.

14.5.1 Documentation, evidence and assessment

- A brief history of the event is documented verbatim including what time, when, where and by whom. Information on the sexual acts which occurred, ejaculation and condom use is elicited. This is in addition to current symptoms, past medical history, medication, contraception and allergies. An examination should be undertaken with sensitivity and in an unhurried manner, with clear documentation of any injuries. Examination of the oral cavity and proctoscopy is undertaken, as indicated by the history.
- If the assault was within the last 7 days management of any injuries sustained may be required. In addition, consideration and discussion about a forensic medical examination to gather evidence is recommended. Forensic examinations are undertaken in Sexual Assault Referral Centres (SARC): swabs for DNA can be taken (see *Table 14.3* for DNA evidence collection timing), injuries documented, and immediate medical care as well as emergency contraception, HIV prophylaxis and hepatitis B vaccination can be provided. SARCs vary across the country and so it is advisable to check on the services offered locally.

Table 14.3 DNA forensic sample timetable

Site	Time up to which DNA can be detected
Vaginal	7 days
Anal	3 days
Oral	2 days
Digital penetration	12 hours

- If an individual presents immediately after the assault they are advised not to shower or bathe, brush their teeth or wash their clothes. All clothes should be kept along with any pads or tampons worn at the time of the assault as they may provide evidence.
- An assessment of psychological wellbeing and for symptoms of post-traumatic stress disorder, if the presentation is later, with particular reference to risk of self-harm and suicide is advisable. In addition, it is important to ascertain if it is safe to allow the individual to go home or if emergency accommodation is required as well as determining if there are any ongoing child or vulnerable adult protection issues.
- Some services undertake baseline STI screens while others wait until 2 weeks after the assault for chlamydia and gonorrhoea, and 3 months for HIV, syphilis and hepatitis B and C. Alternatively serum samples may be taken and saved and only tested after 3 months if any of the repeat blood tests are positive; a negative saved serum may indicate an association between the alleged assault and the acquisition of infection.
- Prophylactic antibiotics can be provided to women with a history of sexual assault; this reduces the need for testing and the chance of missing an infection if the individual defaults from follow-up. However, this approach may result in unnecessary treatment and reduces the potential for partner notification and increases the chance of re-infection if the original infection was from someone other than the assailant.

14.5.2 Hepatitis vaccination

Although the acquisition of hepatitis from sexual assault in the UK is uncommon, vaccination may be given up to 6 weeks after an assault in the following circumstances:
- Assailant known to be hepatitis B carrier.
- Assailant has risk factor(s), for example, intravenous drug users or man who has sex with men.
- Anal assault.
- Trauma and bleeding following the assault.
- Multiple assailants.
- Client wishes to have vaccination.

The vaccination may be given on day 0, 7 and 21 or day 0, at 1 month and at 2 months following the assault. Either regimen is followed by a booster at 1 year.

14.5.3 HIV post-exposure prophylaxis (PEP) following sexual exposure

For individuals presenting within 72 hours of the assault, PEP can be considered. An assessment of the risk of transmission, which is determined from the assailant's likelihood of having HIV and the risk per exposure is undertaken (see *Figure 14.1* and *Table 14.5*). It is recommended that an individual is advised that there is a lack of conclusive data regarding the efficacy of PEP. Its side-effects, the length of treatment (28 days), the importance of adhering to treatment, and the frequency of follow-up should also be discussed. PEP can often be obtained from A&E departments or from sexual health services.

• Assailant from high-risk group. • Background local prevalence of HIV in community. • HIV status of assailant (if known). • Assailant thought to come from a high prevalence area. • Type of assault.   • Assailant stranger versus known. • Presence of other STI(s) in the assaulted individual. • Genital injury. • Multiple assailants. • Multiple risk factors.

Figure 14.1 HIV risk factors.

Prior to commencing PEP, a baseline HIV test is recommended.

- The currently recommended regimen for PEP is raltegravir and Truvada for 28 days. One Truvada tablet (245 mg tenofovir disoproxil (as fumarate) and 200 mg emtricitabine (FTC)) once a day plus one raltegravir tablet (400 mg) twice a day. PEP can be used in conjunction with emergency contraception if indicated.
- If PEP is provided, monitoring is undertaken as indicated in *Table 14.4*. HIV testing is recommended 3 months after the completion of treatment (4 months after the assault). (See *Table 14.4*)

Table 14.4 Recommended monitoring during PEP course and follow-up

	Baseline	14 days	8–12 weeks post-exposure
HIV	✔		✔
Hep B sAg (if no history of vaccination)	✔		✔ Only if not immune
STI testing (as appropriate per local clinic policy)	✔	✔	If further UPSI has taken place
Creatinine	✔	Only if abnormalities at baseline	
Alanine transaminase (ALT)	✔	Only if abnormalities at baseline, Hep B/C co-infected or on Kaletra	
Urinalysis or uPCR	✔	Only if abnormalities at baseline	If abnormalities at baseline or 2 weeks
Pregnancy test	✔	If appropriate	If appropriate

Adapted from *International Journal of STD & AIDS* 2016; April: doi: 10.1177/0956462416641813, with permission from SAGE.

Table 14.5 Situations when PEP is considered

	Source HIV status			
	HIV positive		**Unknown HIV status**	
	HIV viral load unknown / detectable (>200 copies/ml)	HIV viral load undetectable (<200 copies/ml)	From high prevalence country / risk group[1]	From low prevalence country / group
Receptive anal sex	Recommend	Not recommended[2] *Provided source has confirmed HIV viral load <200 c/ml for >6 months*	Recommend	Not recommended
Insertive anal sex	Recommend	Not recommended	Consider[3]	Not recommended
Receptive vaginal sex	Recommend	Not recommended	Consider[3]	Not recommended
Insertive vaginal sex	Consider[4]	Not recommended	Consider[3]	Not recommended
Fellatio with ejaculation[5]	Not recommended	Not recommended	Not recommended	Not recommended
Fellatio without ejaculation[5]	Not recommended	Not recommended	Not recommended	Not recommended
Splash of semen into eye	Not recommended	Not recommended	Not recommended	Not recommended
Cunnilingus	Not recommended	Not recommended	Not recommended	Not recommended
Sharing of injecting equipment[6]	Recommend	Not recommended	Consider	Not recommended
Human bite[7]	Not recommended	Not recommended	Not recommended	Not recommended
Needlestick from a discarded needle in the community			Not recommended	Not recommended

Reproduced from *International Journal of STD & AIDS* 2016; April; doi: 10.1177/0956462416641813 with permission from SAGE.

[1] High prevalence countries or risk groups are those where there is a significant likelihood of the source individual being HIV positive. Within the UK at present, this is likely to be men who have sex with men, intravenous drug users from high-risk countries (see footnote 6) and individuals who have immigrated to the UK from areas of high HIV prevalence, particularly sub-Saharan Africa (high prevalence is >1%). Country-specific HIV prevalence can be found in UNAIDS Gap Report: www.unaids.org/en/resources/campaigns/2014/2014gapreport/gapreport.

[2] The source's viral load must be confirmed with the source's clinic as <200 copies/ml for >6 months. Where there is any uncertainty about results or adherence to ART then PEP should be given after unprotected anal intercourse with an HIV-positive person.

[3] More detailed knowledge of local prevalence of HIV within communities may change these recommendations from Consider to Recommend in areas of particularly high HIV prevalence. Co-factors

that influence the likelihood of transmission should be considered (see *Box 1* in the guidelines at www.bashh.org/documents/PEPSE%202015%20guideline%20final_NICE.pdf).

[4] Co-factors in *Box 1* that influence the likelihood of transmission should be considered.

[5] PEP is not recommended for individuals receiving fellatio i.e. inserting their penis into another's oral cavity. For individuals giving fellatio PEP is not recommended unless HIV seroconversion and/or oropharyngeal trauma / ulceration are present; see notes in guideline cited in footnote 3.

[6] HIV prevalence amongst intravenous drug users varies considerably depending on country of origin and is particularly high in those from eastern Europe and central Asia. Region-specific estimates can be found in the UNAIDS Gap Report: www.unaids.org/sites/default/files/media_asset/05_Peoplewhoinjectdrugs.pdf.

[7] A bite is assumed to constitute breakage of the skin with passage of blood. See notes in guideline cited in footnote 3 about extreme circumstances where PEP could be considered after discussion with a specialist.

14.5.4 Pregnancy following assault

There is approximately a 5% risk of pregnancy following a sexual assault. For individuals not currently using contraception the need for emergency contraception should be considered (see *Chapter 13*). Pregnancy testing is undertaken no earlier than 3 weeks after the sexual assault.

14.5.5 Psychological considerations following sexual assault

Long-term psychological support may be needed for victims of sexual assault because anxiety and depression are common consequences and post-traumatic stress disorder may develop. Assessment of psychological needs can and should be undertaken by any healthcare professional and should include self-harm risk assessment and onward referral as needed. In view of the potential long-term sequelae of sexual assault, if an individual presents to a GUM or integrated sexual health service, letters indicating the reason for the attendance are often sent to the individual's GP with the attendee's consent.

EXAMPLE

A 28 year old school receptionist attends for a contraception discussion at her GPs. She states she has no symptoms but she ended the relationship with her partner of 2 years about a month ago when she discovered he had another sexual partner.

Which questions are you going to ask her? Which investigations are you going to offer and when will you need to repeat any of the investigations?

1. Ask about potential symptoms, including change in vaginal discharge, dysuria, abdominal or pelvic pain, skin changes. Also ask about menstrual history, including last menstrual period, intermenstrual or post-coital bleeding. Ask about current contraception and condom use, previous sexual partner(s), history of previous STIs and blood-borne virus risk assessment.
2. Offer physical examination even in absence of symptoms because infection with, for example, genital warts may be identified.
3. Screening of vagina with NAAT for chlamydia and gonorrhoea, and clotted blood for HIV and syphilis form the main components of a routine asymptomatic screen. If the last sexual contact was more than 3 months ago no further testing will be required. In this particular case HIV and syphilis testing should be repeated 3 months after the last sexual contact.

References

BASHH (2008) *UK National Guidelines for HIV Testing*. BHIVA, BASHH, BIF
[www.bashh.org – accessed May 2023]

BASHH (2012a) *UK National Guidelines on Safer Sex Advice*. Clinical Effectiveness Group BASHH and BHIVA.
[www.bashh.org – accessed May 2023]

BASHH (2012b) *UK National Guidelines on the Management of Adult and Adolescent Complainants of Sexual Assault*. Clinical Effectiveness Group
[www.bashh.org – accessed May 2023]

BASHH (2015) *Summary Guidance on Test for Sexually Transmitted Infection*. Clinical Effectiveness Group.
[www.bashh.org – accessed May 2023]

BASHH (2015) *UK Guideline for the Use of HIV Post-Exposure Prophylaxis Following Sexual Exposure (PEPSE)*
[www.bashh.org/documents/PEPSE%202015%20guideline%20final_NICE.pdf – accessed May 2023]

BASHH (2018) *Guideline for the Management of Infection with* Mycoplasma genitalium. Clinical Effectiveness Group.
[www.bashhguidelines.org/media/1228/mg-ijstdaids.pdf – accessed May 2023]

BASHH/BHIVA (2018) *Guidelines on the Use of HIV Pre-exposure Prophylaxis (PrEP)*
[www.bashhguidelines.org/media/1189/prep-2018.pdf – accessed May 2023]

Chapter 15
Unplanned pregnancy

15.1 Introduction

A recent study estimated that worldwide, 44% of all pregnancies between 2010 and 2014 were unplanned. The same study identified an unintended pregnancy rate between 2010 and 2014 of 27 per 1000 women in northern Europe (women aged 15–44 years). In addition, during this time period 64% of unintended pregnancies ended in abortion in northern Europe.

For some women discovering they are pregnant is an exciting, highly anticipated event. For others it can be associated with mixed emotions including:
- shock that they are actually pregnant
- concern about the responsibility associated with being pregnant
- fear that they are not ready, or are unable to afford a child (or another child)
- anger that they did not choose to be pregnant
- anxiety about being pregnant, concerns about childbirth or how their peers and family will view the pregnancy
- concern that they need to make a decision about the pregnancy and fear they will make the wrong decision
- negative associations with the conception and/or father, particularly in the case of the victims of sexual assault.

The provision of, or access to services to facilitate the management of an unplanned pregnancy is an essential component of any contraception and sexual health service.

Women who become aware of their pregnancy while using hormonal contraception can be reassured that these hormones are not thought to cause harm to the fetus, and they should not be advised to terminate the pregnancy because of this exposure.

For women who intend to continue with their pregnancy, the method of contraception is usually stopped or removed. Women using IUC who are less than 12 weeks' gestation should have the IUC removed, as long as the threads are visible or it can be easily removed from the endocervical canal, regardless of whether the woman decides to continue with the pregnancy or not. Whilst there is a small risk of miscarriage associated with removal, removing the IUC in the first trimester could improve pregnancy outcomes.

For women who do not intend to continue with their pregnancy, if they are using the IMP or injectable they can continue with their method. Women using the CHC or POP can be advised to stop their method and restart it immediately after the abortion.

Support and information are available for women who find that they are pregnant and are not sure what to do. The options include:
- continuing with the pregnancy and keeping the baby, or opting for fostering or adoption
- ending the pregnancy with an abortion.

Discussion with family members, friends, medical and nursing professionals and charitable organizations can provide support and information to facilitate the decision-making process.

15.2 Adoption

- Adoption is an option for women who do not feel able to keep the baby but do not wish or are too late to have an abortion.
- The process of adoption is organized by voluntary adoption agencies and adoption agencies that are part of local councils.
- A birth parent cannot give consent to adoption until their child is at least 6 weeks old.
- Those wishing to adopt undergo an assessment process. A report is then generated and reviewed by an independent adoption panel who make a recommendation to the adoption agency based on the assessment. The adoption panel send their recommendation to the agency, which will then decide whether those wishing to adopt a child are suitable. Once approved, prospective adopters are matched with a child and this match is then reviewed.
- There is a minimum 10-week period of time during which the child must live with the adopters before an Adoption Order can be made.
- The Adoption Order is the legal procedure in which the parental responsibility for a child is transferred to the adopter, at which time they become the child's legal parent.
- More information can be found at CoramBAAF adoption and fostering academy (https://corambaaf.org.uk) and from local social services.

15.3 Abortion

- The Abortion Act (1967) makes abortion legal where the pregnancy is terminated by a registered medical practitioner and, except in emergencies, where two registered medical practitioners are of the opinion formed in good faith that one of the lawful grounds in the Act is met (see *Figure 15.1*). This legislation applies to England, Scotland and Wales. See *Section 15.7* for the legal situation in Northern Ireland and the Republic of Ireland.
- In response to the Covid-19 pandemic, Ministers in England, Scotland and Wales granted temporary permission for early medical abortion treatment to be received by post following a telemedical consultation. On 30 March 2022, following a Parliamentary vote in favour of an amendment to the Health and Care Bill, the temporary approval allowing home use of both pills (mifepristone and the second component, misoprostol) for early medical abortions was made permanent in England and Wales. In May 2022, the Scottish Government confirmed that early medical abortion at home, when clinically appropriate, would continue long-term. In March 2023, an evaluation in Scotland reported back supporting the effectiveness and acceptability of at-home abortion.
- Legal abortion is a safe way to end a pregnancy. It is the most common gynaecological procedure undertaken in Great Britain and by the age of 45 one-third of women will have had an abortion.

- Abortion rates continue to rise in England, Scotland and Wales.
- The majority of abortions occur at early gestations. In Scotland 73% of all abortions were at less than 9 weeks' gestation and in England and Wales 80% of abortions were performed under 10 weeks' gestation.
- In the UK medical abortion is the most common method of terminating a pregnancy. In Scotland in 2018 nearly 30% of all medical abortions involved self-administration of misoprostol at home.
- Although the structure of abortion services varies from area to area, all women considering this option should have access to care and services of a uniformly high quality.
- Under the current commissioning structure, in England abortions are commissioned by clinical commissioning groups. A full range of services including a choice of medical and surgical procedures for all gestations, up to the legal limit of 24 weeks of gestation, should be provided either directly or through a referral pathway.
- Services are provided by the NHS or independent providers such as Marie Stopes International (MSI) or British Pregnancy Advisory Service (BPAS). In accordance with the 1967 Abortion Act, an abortion can only be carried out in locations approved by the Secretary of State for Health.
- Generally abortion services are widely accessible and take referrals from a number of sources including general practitioners, sexual health services and self-referral (ideally via a centralized telephone system).
- Once a woman makes the decision that she would like to proceed with an abortion there should be minimal delay. An initial assessment appointment is ideally offered within 1 week of the request. The time from initially seeing the provider and making a decision to the abortion taking place should ideally be less than a week.
- Importantly, a woman can cancel or delay appointments or the procedure at any point if she wishes to.

15.3.1 Pre-abortion assessment

- This assessment can be undertaken as a face-to-face consultation or via telephone or video call, and may be offered in a range of settings including hospital and community services, depending on local need.
- Within the consultation the following should be documented:
  - reasons why the unplanned pregnancy may have occurred and why the woman is requesting an abortion
  - details of the past menstrual history, including last menstrual period and cycle
  - previous contraceptive methods used and problems with these methods
  - contraceptive plans for the future
  - past medical history, including obstetric history, with the aim of identifying relevant acute or chronic medical conditions which may require specialist care (robust referral pathway to specialist services are required)

- ○ social and relationship history, with particular reference to domestic violence, coercion or exploitation and safeguarding issues.
- Pregnancy should be confirmed. Although an ultrasound scan is not essential it is increasingly being used to assess gestation and to confirm that the pregnancy is within the uterine cavity.
- Discuss pregnancy options, including fostering and adoption.
- Identify women who require more support in the decision-making process and refer on as needed to appropriate services.
- Methods of abortion should be discussed and the procedures explained, including potential adverse effects and complications. As well as the symptoms likely to be experienced both during and after the abortion (e.g. menstrual-like cramps, pain and bleeding), that products of conception may be seen (medical only), approximately how long it will take for the abortion to be completed, how they will know when it is complete, which pain management options will be made available, follow-up care and the range of potential emotions experienced following the abortion. This should be supported by written information. This approach enables women to select the correct choice of method for them.
- STI screening should be undertaken in at-risk groups along with standard assessment of VTE risk and rhesus status.
- Finally, consent for the chosen procedure is obtained and the HSA1 form in England and Wales or Certificate A in Scotland is completed by two doctors indicating in good faith the grounds for performing the abortion (see *Figure 15.1*). It is not legally essential for either or both doctors to see the patient before the HSA1 form or Certificate A is completed; however, they must review each case and document in the clinical notes the grounds for performing the abortion, before the abortion is performed. **C** is the most common ground for performing an abortion (see *Figure 15.1*).

A	Continuance of the pregnancy would involve risk to the life of the pregnant woman greater than if the pregnancy were terminated
B	Termination is necessary to prevent grave permanent injury to the physical or mental health of the pregnant woman
C	The pregnancy has NOT exceeded its 24th week and continuance of the pregnancy would involve risk, greater than if the pregnancy were terminated, of injury to the physical or mental health of the pregnant woman
D	The pregnancy has NOT exceeded its 24th week and continuance of the pregnancy would involve risk, greater than if the pregnancy were terminated, of injury to the physical or mental health of any existing child(ren) of the family of the pregnant woman
E	There is a substantial risk that if the child were born it would suffer from such physical or mental abnormalities as to be seriously handicapped

Figure 15.1 Grounds for abortion in the UK.

15.3.2 Abortion procedures

- Providers should ideally give a choice of medical and surgical abortion, irrespective of gestation.
- The options for method of abortion are determined by gestation and the wishes of the woman in attendance (see *Figure 15.2*).
- While the majority of procedures are undertaken as day cases, certain circumstances such as medical problems, social indications, geographical factors or individual choice may necessitate an in-patient stay.

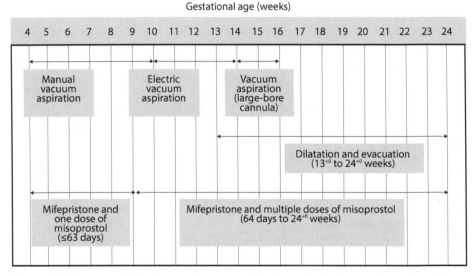

Figure 15.2 Summary of abortion methods appropriate for use in abortion services in the UK by gestational age (in weeks). Figure adapted and reproduced with permission from the Royal College of Obstetricians and Gynaecologists.

Medical abortion

Medical abortion (with mifepristone and misoprostol) is *licensed* for the provision of abortion up to 9 weeks and from 13 weeks to 23 weeks and 6 days. However, in practice it is provided at all gestations. Medical abortions may occur within a hospital or clinic setting, or in an individual's home.

- Medical abortion is often a two-stage process:
  - initially, mifepristone is administered orally; it is a steroid with a similar structure to progesterone which blocks the action of progesterone on the uterus and cervix. It promotes uterine contractions following the administration of misoprostol. If vomiting occurs within one hour of taking mifepristone an individual should be advised to return to the clinic for a repeat dose of mifepristone
  - 24–48 hours after the first stage, misoprostol is administered; it causes uterine contraction and expulsion of the products of conception

- Up to and including 9+0 weeks' gestation women may have the option of taking oral mifepristone and vaginal misoprostol at the same time. The risk of ongoing pregnancy may be higher and it may take longer for the bleeding and pain to start than with the 2-stage process.
- In later gestations (10+1 to 23+6 weeks), if an interval of less than 36 hours between mifepristone and misoprostol is chosen, women need to be aware that it may take a longer time from taking the first misoprostol dose to complete the abortion. Following the first dose, further doses of misoprostol may be administered at 3-hourly intervals, via vaginal, sublingual or buccal routes until expulsion.
- The options for administration of misoprostol for early medical abortion (less than 10 weeks' gestation) include:
  ◦ mifepristone and misoprostol can be sent to a woman's home or collected and self-administered at home
  ◦ self-administration of misoprostol at home (up to and including 9 weeks and 6 days' gestation)
  ◦ misoprostol administered in hospital or clinic and the woman remains in the clinic or hospital until the products of conception are seen
  ◦ misoprostol administered in hospital or clinic where a woman remains for a short time, following which she may choose to leave and complete the abortion at home
- Above 21 weeks of gestation, the abortion is preceded by fetocide, most commonly achieved by injecting potassium chloride under ultrasound guidance.
- Early medical abortion (before 9 weeks of gestation) is very effective, with a failure rate of less than 1 in 200.
- Symptoms experienced during medical abortion include cramping abdominal pain, bleeding, nausea, vomiting, diarrhoea, flushes and sweats and dizziness.

Surgical abortion

Surgical abortion can be carried out at all gestations up to 23 weeks and 6 days:
- a suction termination can be performed up to 13 weeks
- dilatation and evacuation (D&E) of the uterus is carried out in later gestations because the products are too large to be removed intact through the cervix and are therefore removed piecemeal; this procedure is normally performed under ultrasound guidance.

Under 13 weeks of gestation, there are two methods of surgical abortion depending on local availability.
- Manual vacuum aspiration (MVA) is performed under local anaesthetic or conscious sedation. A plastic cannula is introduced through the cervix and an aspirator attached. The vacuum is released and uterine evacuation accomplished.
- Electronic vacuum aspiration (EVA) is performed under general anaesthetic. Appropriate cervical dilatation is undertaken, with graduated dilators if needed, then the suction curette is introduced through the cervix and suction applied; the products are removed in a closed system until complete evacuation of the uterus is achieved.

Cervical priming, for example 400 micrograms of sublingual misoprostol an hour before the abortion and 400 micrograms of vaginal misoprostol 3 hours before the abortion reduces the risk of cervical trauma and for MVA may remove the need for dilatation. At later gestations osmotic dilators may be used prior to the procedure.

15.3.3 Following the abortion

- Antibiotic prophylaxis is not routinely offered to women having a medical abortion. Antibiotic prophylaxis is offered to women having a surgical abortion. NICE (2019) advises doxycycline 100 mg twice a day for 3 days, and while acknowledging that there may be circumstances in which metronidazole is indicated, it should not be routinely prescribed.
- Rhesus status is determined prior to an abortion. Anti-D prophylaxis is offered to women who are rhesus D negative and are having an abortion after 10+0 weeks' gestation. Anti-D prophylaxis may be beneficial for women having a surgical abortion up to and including 10+0 weeks' gestation.
- In England and Wales an HSA4 form is completed by the practitioner undertaking the abortion, either online or as a paper copy, and sent to the Chief Medical Officer within 14 days of the abortion. In Scotland a notification form (the yellow form) is completed by the practitioner undertaking the abortion and returned to the Chief Medical Officer of Scotland within 7 days of the abortion.
- When completing the Abortion Notification the address of treatment with prostaglandin must be the woman's home/residence for those women who choose an abortion at home; likewise the date of treatment with prostaglandin should be recorded as the date on which the patient was advised to self-administer the misoprostol.
- Pregnancy remains should always be managed respectfully. Disposal is by cremation or burial and is generally organized by the hospital or clinic performing the abortion. However, women may choose to make their own arrangements; if they do, the remains are kept in suitable storage and collection recorded in accordance with local protocols. Women who have an abortion at home are generally provided with the option of bringing the products to hospital for disposal.

15.4 Complications

Abortion is a safe procedure with major complications rare at all gestations (see *Table 15.1*). Estimated complication rates are 1–2 per 100 abortions. It is difficult to truly determine the rate, partly due to lack of standardization of reporting criteria and partly because women experiencing complications often present to other healthcare providers.

15.5 Post-abortion contraception

Provision of contraception immediately following abortion is key to reducing further unplanned pregnancies. Wherever possible the chosen method should be started

Table 15.1 Complications of surgical and medical abortion

Complication	Rate
Uterine perforation (surgical only)	1–4 per 1000
Haemorrhage	1–4 per 1000
Cervix trauma (surgical only)	1 per 100
Infection	1 per 10
Retained products of conception	5 per 100
Failure of procedure to end pregnancy	1 per 100
Anaesthetic	Rare
Psychological consequences	Currently not quantified
Infertility	No proven association

immediately following the abortion. Where the requested method is not available a bridging method can be provided.

- Most contraceptive methods including CHC, POP, injectable, implant and IUC can be started immediately or soon after a medical or surgical abortion.
- Women who choose the injectable method can be given their injection at the same time as the mifepristone, although there is a small increased risk of an ongoing pregnancy.
- A diaphragm can be fitted 4–6 weeks after abortion.
- Sterilization is ideally undertaken 3 months after an abortion to allow time to consider this permanent choice.

Ideally, if a chosen method of contraception is not available within the abortion service there should referral pathways in place to local sexual health services or general practitioners.

15.6 Aftercare

- After an abortion a 24-hour telephone number should be provided to women so that they can access help or discuss any concerns.
- Women should contact abortion services or their general practitioner post-procedure if they have a temperature >37.5°C, have persisting abdominal pain, prolonged heavy bleeding (heavier than first day of normal period or soaking 2 maxi pads in an hour for more than 2 hours), abdominal tenderness or abnormal vaginal discharge.
- Women are generally advised that routine follow-up is not needed. Pregnancy symptoms resolve within 3 days of the abortion and their next period will occur within 4–6 weeks.
- Women who have taken misoprostol at home need to contact their provider if they do not bleed within 24 hours of receiving misoprostol or they do not take the misoprostol as advised. Women who had their abortion at home may have face-to-face or remote follow-up. They are provided with a multi-level or low sensitivity pregnancy test which is undertaken 2 weeks after the procedure, to exclude an ongoing pregnancy.

15.7 Legal situation in Ireland

15.7.1 Northern Ireland

- For over half a century the law on abortion in Northern Ireland has been much more restrictive than that in the rest of the UK.
- However, on 9 July 2019 an amendment was successfully attached to the Government's Northern Ireland (Executive Formation) Act requiring the Government to liberalize abortion law in Northern Ireland if the Assembly did not reconvene by 21 October 2019.
- On 22 October 2019 abortion was decriminalised in Northern Ireland. This means that no further police investigations or prosecutions may be carried out under the old law (for offences relating to Sections 58 and 59 of the Offences Against the Person Act 1861). It also means that any current or pending prosecutions will be cancelled.
- Section 25 (1) of the Criminal Justice Act (Northern Ireland) 1945 is, for now, still in effect. This means that abortions "where the foetus is capable of being born alive" will still be unlawful.
- The UK Government is now required to fulfil its obligations under the Northern Ireland (Executive Formation etc) Act 2019. Currently consultation documents containing proposed legislative and regulatory frameworks for the provision of abortion services are being considered. The framework will reportedly be based upon recommendations made in the Committee on the Elimination of Discrimination against Women (CEDAW) 2018 report. The new frameworks are to be in place by 31 March 2020, when local services will take over the provision of abortion in Northern Ireland. The newly reconvened Assembly will be involved in the generation of the frameworks.
- Until services are in place in Northern Ireland, abortions will be provided in England via a centralized booking service. All aspects of the service are funded including travel and, where required, overnight accommodation.
- At the time of writing we do not know if the CEDAW recommendations will be implemented or to what extent the regulations put in place by March 2020 will affect access and availability regarding gestation, nor the certification or notification requirements.

15.7.2 Republic of Ireland

- On 25 May 2018 the people of the Republic of Ireland voted to repeal the Eighth Amendment of the constitution of Ireland, removing the ban on abortion.
- The Health (Regulation of Termination of Pregnancy) Act 2018 defines the circumstances and means by which abortion can be legally performed in Ireland.
- Abortion services commenced on 1 January 2019.
- This Act permits abortions to be carried out up to 12 weeks of pregnancy.
- Abortion services are provided by GPs, family planning clinics, women's health clinics and hospitals. Women over 9 weeks' gestation and those with medical complications are provided with abortion care in a hospital setting.

- A woman requesting an abortion is certified as being less than 12 weeks' gestation either by dates or ultrasound scan if indicated. Following this there is a 3-day wait. Legally there must be at least 3 days from certification to having the abortion. The delay gives women time to decide that they definitely want to go ahead with the abortion.
- After 12 weeks it is possible to access abortion care in Ireland if there is a risk of serious harm or a risk to the life of the pregnant person. It is also possible to access abortion care if there has been a diagnosis of fatal fetal abnormality.
- Women who are over 12 weeks of pregnancy can currently travel to Great Britain to access abortion care. The potential impact of the UK's intention to leave the EU on rights and costs associated with travelling to Great Britain is as yet unknown.

15.8 Myths and misconceptions

- **You will not be able to become pregnant again after having an abortion** – this is not true. Well-designed studies show no connection between abortion and future fertility problems. There is less evidence investigating repeat or second-trimester abortion but current research indicates no association in the absence of complications. Also there is currently no proven association between abortion and subsequent ectopic pregnancy or placenta praevia or breast cancer or mental health conditions.
- **Abortions can weaken the cervix making premature delivery of a baby more common following such a procedure** – this is not true. There was a link 20–30 years ago when there was a 10–20% increased risk, but with modern abortion methods (particularly medical) abortion data from 2000 onwards shows no evidence of an association between abortion and premature delivery in subsequent pregnancies.

EXAMPLE

A 19 year old attends your practice with a positive pregnancy test. Her last period was 7 weeks ago.

What additional information would you need and what are her options?

1. Is the pregnancy planned and how does she feel about being pregnant?
2. Document details of menstrual cycle, current contraception, medical history and social history.
3. Discuss all options available, including continuing with the pregnancy and keeping the baby or placing the child in foster care or for adoption, or abortion.
4. If abortion is requested by this 19 year old, referral/self-referral to an abortion service should be expedited. At this clinic an assessment is undertaken.
5. Both medical and surgical abortion may be discussed and the most appropriate method selected by the individual.
6. Contraception after abortion should be covered pre-abortion and commenced immediately after the procedure or with minimal delay.

- **Abortions cause long-term psychological harm for most women** – there is no well-conducted research to support this. Women with an unwanted pregnancy are at risk of mental health problems, but a woman with an unwanted pregnancy is equally as likely to have mental health problems from experiencing an abortion as she is from giving birth.

References

Bearak, J. *et al.* (2018) Global, regional, and subregional trends in unintended pregnancy and its outcomes from 1990 to 2014: estimates from a Bayesian hierarchical model. *The Lancet Global Health*, **6(4)**: 380–389.

Committee on the Elimination of Discrimination against Women (2018) *Report of the Inquiry concerning the United Kingdom of Great Britain and Northern Ireland under Article 8 of the Optional Protocol to the Convention on the Elimination of All Forms of Discrimination against Women*
[http://tbinternet.ohchr.org/Treaties/CEDAW/Shared%20Documents/GBR/INT_CEDAW_ITB_GBR_8637_E.pdf – accessed May 2023]

Department of Health (2014) *Guidance in Relation to Requirements of the Abortion Act 1967*
[www.gov.uk/government/uploads/system/uploads/attachment_data/file/313459/20140509_-_Abortion_Guidance_Document.pdf – accessed May 2023]

Department of Health and Social Care (2023) *Abortion Statistics, England and Wales: 2021*
[www.gov.uk/government/statistics/abortion-statistics-for-england-and-wales-2021/abortion-statistics-england-and-wales-2021 – accessed May 2023]

HM Government (2019) *Child Adoption*
[www.gov.uk/child-adoption – accessed May 2023]

Human Tissue Authority (2015) *Guidance on the Disposal of Pregnancy Remains Following Pregnancy Loss or Termination*
[https://content.hta.gov.uk/sites/default/files/2021-06/Guidance%20on%20the%20disposal%20of%20pregnacy%20remains.pdf – accessed May 2023]

Information Services Division Scotland (2019) *Termination of Pregnancy* (year ending Dec 2018)
[www.isdscotland.org/Health-Topics/Sexual-Health/Publications/2019-05-28/2019-05-28-Terminations-2018-Report.pdf – accessed May 2023]

NICE (2019) NG140 *Abortion Care*
[www.nice.org.uk/guidance/ng140/resources/abortion-care-pdf-66141773098693 – accessed May 2023]

RCOG (2011) *The Care of Women Requesting Induced Abortion* (Evidence-based Guideline Number 7)
[www.rcog.org.uk/globalassets/documents/guidelines/abortion-guideline_web_1.pdf – accessed May 2023]

RCOG (2015, updated 2022) *Best Practice in Abortion Care* (Best Practice Paper No. 2)
[www.rcog.org.uk/media/geify5bx/abortion-care-best-practice-paper-april-2022.pdf – accessed May 2023]

RCOG (2019) *Clinical Guidelines for Early Medical Abortion at Home – England*
[www.rcog.org.uk/en/guidelines-research-services/guidelines/early-medical-abortion-home-england – accessed May 2023]

Appendix

Summary of the UKMEC for contraceptive use

Reproduced under licence from FSRH. Copyright © Faculty of Sexual and Reproductive Healthcare 2006 to 2016. The FSRH is the largest UK professional membership organization in sexual and reproductive health working to shape better sexual health for all (www.fsrh.org). The UKMEC summary table was amended in September 2019; changes are shown here in bold.

UKMEC Categories:
1 = no restriction for use
2 = can generally be used but with careful follow-up
3 = not usually recommended but may be used after expert clinical judgement and/or referral to a contraceptive specialist
4 = use poses an unacceptable health risk

UKMEC SUMMARY TABLE HORMONAL AND INTRAUTERINE CONTRACEPTION						
Cu-IUD = Copper-bearing intrauterine device; LNG-IUS = Levonorgestrel-releasing intrauterine system; IMP = Progestogen-only implant; DMPA = Progestogen-only injectable: depot medroxyprogesterone acetate; POP = Progestogen-only pill; CHC = Combined hormonal contraception						
CONDITION	**Cu-IUD**	**LNG-IUS**	**IMP**	**DMPA**	**POP**	**CHC**
	I = Initiation, C = Continuation					
PERSONAL CHARACTERISTICS AND REPRODUCTIVE HISTORY						
Pregnancy	NA	NA	NA	NA	NA	NA
Age	Menarche to <20=2, ≥20=1	Menarche to <20=2, ≥20=1	After menarche = 1	Menarche to <18=2, 18–45=1, >45=2	After menarche = 1	Menarche to <40=1, ≥40=2
Parity						
a) Nulliparous	1	1	1	1	1	1
b) Parous	1	1	1	1	1	1
Breastfeeding						
a) 0 to <6 weeks postpartum	See below		1	2	1	4
b) ≥6 weeks to <6 months (primarily breastfeeding)			1	1	1	2
c) ≥6 months postpartum			1	1	1	1
Postpartum (in non-breastfeeding women)						
a) 0 to <3 weeks						
(i) With other risk factors for VTE	See below		1	2	1	4
(ii) Without other risk factors			1	2	1	3
b) 3 to <6 weeks						
(i) With other risk factors for VTE	See below		1	2	1	3
(ii) Without other risk factors			1	1	1	2
c) ≥6 weeks			1	1	1	1

CONDITION	Cu-IUD	LNG-IUS	IMP	DMPA	POP	CHC
	I = Initiation, C = Continuation					
Postpartum (in breastfeeding or non-breastfeeding women, including post-caesarean section)						
a) 0 to <48 hours	1	1				
b) 48 hours to <4 weeks	3	3		See above		
c) ≥4 weeks	1	1				
d) Postpartum sepsis	4	4				
Post-abortion						
a) First trimester	1	1	1	1	1	1
b) Second trimester	2	2	1	1	1	1
c) Post-abortion sepsis	4	4	1	1	1	1
Past ectopic pregnancy	1	1	1	1	1	1
History of pelvic surgery	1	1	1	1	1	1
Smoking						
a) Age <35 years	1	1	1	1	1	2
b) Age ≥35 years						
(i) <15 cigarettes/day	1	1	1	1	1	3
(ii) ≥15 cigarettes/day	1	1	1	1	1	4
(iii) Stopped smoking <1 year	1	1	1	1	1	3
(iv) Stopped smoking ≥1 year	1	1	1	1	1	2
Obesity						
a) BMI ≥30–34 kg/m²	1	1	1	1	1	2
b) BMI ≥35 kg/m²	1	1	1	1	1	3
History of bariatric surgery						
a) With BMI <30 kg/m²	1	1	1	1	1	1
b) With BMI ≥30–34 kg/m²	1	1	1	1	1	2
c) With BMI ≥35 kg/m²	1	1	1	1	1	3
Organ transplant						
a) Complicated: graft failure (acute or chronic), rejection, cardiac allograft vasculopathy	I C / 3 2	I C / 3 2	2	2	2	3
b) Uncomplicated	2	2	2	2	2	2
CARDIOVASCULAR DISEASE (CVD)						
Multiple risk factors for CVD (such as smoking, diabetes, hypertension, obesity and dyslipidaemias)	1	2	2	3	2	3

CONDITION	Cu-IUD	LNG-IUS	IMP	DMPA	POP	CHC
	I = Initiation, C = Continuation					
Hypertension						
a) Adequately controlled hypertension	1	1	1	2	1	3
b) Consistently elevated BP levels (properly taken measurements)						
(i) Systolic >140–159 mmHg or diastolic >90–99 mmHg	1	1	1	1	1	3
(ii) Systolic ≥160 mmHg or diastolic ≥100 mmHg	1	1	1	2	1	4
c) Vascular disease	1	2	2	3	2	4
History of high BP during pregnancy	1	1	1	1	1	2
Current and history of ischaemic heart disease	1	I 2 / C 3	I 2 / C 3	3	I 2 / C 3	4
Stroke (history of cerebrovascular accident, including TIA)	1	I 2 / C 3	I 2 / C 3	3	I 2 / C 3	4
Known dyslipidaemias	1	2	2	2	2	2
Venous thromboembolism (VTE)						
a) History of VTE	1	2	2	2	2	4
b) Current VTE (on anticoagulants)	1	2	2	2	2	4
c) Family history of VTE						
(i) First-degree relative age <45 years	1	1	1	1	1	3
(ii) First-degree relative age ≥45 years	1	1	1	1	1	2
d) Major surgery						
(i) With prolonged immobilisation	1	2	2	2	2	4
(ii) Without prolonged immobilisation	1	1	1	1	1	2
e) Minor surgery without immobilisation	1	1	1	1	1	1
f) Immobility (unrelated to surgery) (e.g. wheelchair use, debilitating illness)	1	1	1	1	1	3
Superficial venous thrombosis						
a) Varicose veins	1	1	1	1	1	1
b) Superficial venous thrombosis	1	1	1	1	1	2

CONDITION	Cu-IUD	LNG-IUS	IMP	DMPA	POP	CHC
	I = Initiation, C = Continuation					
Known thrombogenic mutations (e.g. factor V Leiden, prothrombin mutation, protein S, protein C and antithrombin deficiencies)	1	2	2	2	2	4
Valvular and congenital heart disease						
a) Uncomplicated	1	1	1	1	1	2
b) Complicated (e.g. pulmonary hypertension, history of subacute bacterial endocarditis)	2	2	1	1	1	4
Cardiomyopathy						
a) Normal cardiac function	1	1	1	1	1	2
b) Impaired cardiac function	2	2	2	2	2	4
Cardiac arrhythmias						
a) Atrial fibrillation	1	2	2	2	2	4
b) Known long QT syndrome	I 3 / C 1	I 3 / C 1	1	2	1	2
NEUROLOGICAL CONDITIONS						
Headaches						
a) Non-migrainous (mild or severe)	1	1	1	1	1	I 1 / C 2
b) Migraine without aura, at any age	1	2	2	2	I 1 / C 2	I 2 / C 3
c) Migraine with aura, at any age	1	2	2	2	2	4
d) History (≥5 years ago) of migraine with aura, any age	1	2	2	2	2	3
Idiopathic intracranial hypertension (IIH)	1	1	1	1	1	2
Epilepsy	1	1	1	1	1	1
Taking anti-epileptic drugs	Certain anti-epileptic drugs have the potential to affect the bioavailability of steroid hormones in hormonal contraception. For up-to-date information on the potential drug interactions between hormonal contraception and anti-epileptic drugs, please refer to the online drug interaction checker available on **Stockley's Interaction Checker website (www.medicinescomplete.com/mc/alerts/current/drug-interactions.htm)**.					
DEPRESSIVE DISORDERS						
Depressive disorders	1	1	1	1	1	1

CONDITION	Cu-IUD	LNG-IUS	IMP	DMPA	POP	CHC
	I = Initiation, C = Continuation					
BREAST AND REPRODUCTIVE TRACT CONDITIONS						
Vaginal bleeding patterns						
a) Irregular pattern without heavy bleeding	1	1	2	2	2	1
b) Heavy or prolonged bleeding (includes regular and irregular patterns)	2	I 1 / C 2	2	2	2	1
Unexplained vaginal bleeding (suspicious for serious condition) before evaluation	I 4 / C 2	I 4 / C 2	3	3	2	2
Endometriosis	2	1	1	1	1	1
Benign ovarian tumours (including cysts)	1	1	1	1	1	1
Severe dysmenorrhoea	2	1	1	1	1	1
Gestational trophoblastic disease (GTD)						
a) Undetectable hCG levels	1	1	1	1	1	1
b) Decreasing hCG levels	3	3	1	1	1	1
c) Persistently elevated hCG levels or malignant disease	4	4	1	1	1	1
Cervical ectropion	1	1	1	1	1	1
Cervical intraepithelial neoplasia (CIN)	1	2	1	2	1	2
Cervical cancer						
a) Awaiting treatment	I 4 / C 2	I 4 / C 2	2	2	1	2
b) Radical trachelectomy	3	3	2	2	1	2
Breast conditions						
a) Undiagnosed mass/breast symptoms	1	2	2	2	2	I 3 / C 2
b) Benign breast conditions	1	1	1	1	1	1
c) Family history of breast cancer	1	1	1	1	1	1
d) Carriers of known gene mutations associated with breast cancer (e.g. BRCA1/ BRCA2)	1	2	2	2	2	3
e) Breast cancer						
(i) Current breast cancer	1	4	4	4	4	4
(ii) Past breast cancer	1	3	3	3	3	3

CONDITION	Cu-IUD		LNG-IUS		IMP	DMPA	POP	CHC
	I = Initiation, C = Continuation							
Endometrial cancer	**I**	**C**	**I**	**C**	1	1	1	1
	4	2	4	2				
Ovarian cancer	1		1		1	1	1	1
Uterine fibroids								
a) Without distortion of the uterine cavity	1		1		1	1	1	1
b) With distortion of the uterine cavity	3		3		1	1	1	1
Anatomical abnormalities								
a) Distorted uterine cavity	3		3					
b) Other abnormalities	2		2					
Pelvic inflammatory disease (PID)								
a) Past PID (assuming no current risk factor for STIs)	1		1		1	1	1	1
b) Current PID	**I**	**C**	**I**	**C**	1	1	1	1
	4	2	4	2				
Sexually transmitted infections (STIs)								
a) Chlamydial infection (current)	**I**	**C**	**I**	**C**				
(i) Symptomatic	4	2	4	2	1	1	1	1
(ii) Asymptomatic	3	2	3	2	1	1	1	1
b) Purulent cervicitis or gonorrhoea (current)	4	2	4	2	1	1	1	1
c) Other current STIs (excluding HIV & hepatitis)	2		2		1	1	1	1
d) Vaginitis (including *Trichomonas vaginalis* and bacterial vaginosis) (current)	2		2		1	1	1	1
e) Increased risk for STIs	2		2		1	1	1	1
HIV INFECTION								
HIV infection	The following bold entries are additions to the UKMEC in 2019							
a) High risk of HIV infection	**1**		**1**		1	1	1	1
b) HIV infected								
(i) CD4 count ≥200 cells/mm³	2		2		1	1	1	1
(ii) CD4 count <200 cells/mm³	**I**	**C**	**I**	**C**	1	1	1	1
	3	2	3	2				

CONDITION	Cu-IUD	LNG-IUS	IMP	DMPA	POP	CHC
	I = Initiation, C = Continuation					
c) Taking antiretroviral (ARV) drugs	Certain ARV drugs have the potential to affect the bioavailability of steroid hormones in hormonal contraception. For up-to-date information on the potential drug interactions between hormonal contraception and ARV drugs, please refer to the online HIV drugs interaction checker (www.hiv-druginteractions.org/interactions.aspx).					
OTHER INFECTIONS						
Tuberculosis						
a) Non-pelvic	1	1	1	1	1	1
b) Pelvic	I 4 C 3	I 4 C 3	1	1	1	1
ENDOCRINE CONDITIONS						
Diabetes						
a) History of gestational disease	1	1	1	1	1	1
b) Non-vascular disease						
(i) Non-insulin dependent	1	2	2	2	2	2
(ii) Insulin dependent	1	2	2	2	2	2
c) Nephropathy/retinopathy/ neuropathy	1	2	2	2	2	3
d) Other vascular disease	1	2	2	2	2	3
Thyroid disorders						
a) Simple goitre	1	1	1	1	1	1
b) Hyperthyroid	1	1	1	1	1	1
c) Hypothyroid	1	1	1	1	1	1
GASTROINTESTINAL CONDITIONS						
Gallbladder disease						
a) Symptomatic						
(i) Treated by cholecystectomy	1	2	2	2	2	2
(ii) Medically treated	1	2	2	2	2	3
(iii) Current	1	2	2	2	2	3
b) Asymptomatic	1	2	2	2	2	2
History of cholestasis						
a) Pregnancy related	1	1	1	1	1	2
b) Past COC related	1	2	2	2	2	3
Viral hepatitis						
a) Acute or flare	1	1	1	1	1	I 3 C 2
b) Carrier	1	1	1	1	1	1

CONDITION	Cu-IUD	LNG-IUS	IMP	DMPA	POP	CHC
	I = Initiation, C = Continuation					
c) Chronic	1	1	1	1	1	1
Cirrhosis						
a) Mild (compensated without complications)	1	1	1	1	1	1
b) Severe (decompensated)	1	3	3	3	3	4
Liver tumours						
a) Benign						
(i) Focal nodular hyperplasia	1	2	2	2	2	2
(ii) Hepatocellular adenoma	1	3	3	3	3	4
b) Malignant (hepatocellular carcinoma)	1	3	3	3	3	4
Inflammatory bowel disease (including Crohn's disease and ulcerative colitis)	1	1	1	1	2	2
ANAEMIAS						
Thalassaemia	2	1	1	1	1	1
Sickle cell disease	2	1	1	1	1	2
Iron deficiency anaemia	2	1	1	1	1	1
RHEUMATIC DISEASES						
Rheumatoid arthritis	1	2	2	2	2	2
Systemic lupus erythematosus (SLE)						
a) No antiphospholipid antibodies	1	2	2	2	2	2
b) Positive antiphospholipid antibodies	1	2	2	2	2	4
Positive antiphospholipid antibodies	1	2	2	2	2	4
DRUG INTERACTIONS						
Taking medication	See section on drug interactions with hormonal contraception.					

Index

Bold indicates main entry
Italic indicates a figure or table